Oral Health for the Orthodontic Patient

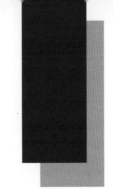

Oral Health for the Orthodontic Patient

Siegward D. Heintze, Dr Med Dent
Department of Pediatric Dentistry
Humbolt University, Berlin

Paul-Georg Jost-Brinkmann, Dr Med Dent
Department of Orthodontics
Humbolt University, Berlin

Christian Finke, Dr Med Dent
Department of Pediatric Dentistry
Humbolt University, Berlin

Rainer-Reginald Miethke, Prof Dr Med Dent
Department of Orthodontics
Humbolt University, Berlin

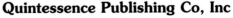

Quintessence Publishing Co, Inc
Chicago, Berlin, London, Tokyo, Paris, Barcelona, São Paulo, Moscow,
Prague, and Warsaw

quintessence
books

Library of Congress Cataloging-in-Publication Data

Oral health for the orthodontic patient / Siegward D. Heintze ... [et al.].
    p.   cm.
  Includes bibliographical references and index.
  ISBN 0–86715-295-8
  1. Periodontitis—Prevention.   2. Periodontitis—Patients—Care.   3. Mouth—Care and
hygiene.   4. Dental health education.   5. Teeth—Care and hygiene.   6. Orthodontics.
I. Heintze, Siegward D.
  RK450.P4073   1998
  617.6'32—dc21   98-8476
                                                                           CIP

quinte//ence
book/

© 1999 Quintessence Publishing Co, Inc

Quintessence Publishing Co, Inc
551 Kimberly Drive
Carol Stream, Illinois 60188

Editor: Cheryl Anderson-Wiedenbeck
Production: Michael Shanahan
Cover design: Michael Shanahan

Printed in Hong Kong

Contents

Chapter 5 *Pharmaceutical Adjuvants for Preventing Caries and Periodontal Disease*

Chapter 6 *Systematic Program for Preventing Caries and Periodontal Disease in Orthodontic Patients*

Introduction

The frequency of orthodontic treatment is increasing. For example, more than half of the adolescents in Germany are being treated orthodontically today, in contrast to the low percentage who had such therapy in the 1950s (Kess et al 1991). In the United States 9.4% of the 8- to 11-year-olds and 24.9% of the 12- to 17-year-olds received orthodontic treatment, with a higher percentage of females than males and more white non-Hispanics than blacks or Mexican Americans (Brunelle et al 1996). The reasons for this increase include not only an actual increase in the incidence of malpositioned teeth and jaws in industrialized nations (Ghafari et al 1989, Heikinheimo 1990, Varella 1990) but also an improved financial situation and a more demanding sense of esthetics by parents and children (Shaw et al 1980). Approximately one fourth of those interviewed in a study of a representative German population (Kess et al 1991) expressed dissatisfaction with the position and appearance of their teeth. Adolescents, in particular, claimed to be teased by their schoolmates and avoided being photographed with their teeth showing.

Ideally, orthodontic treatment is a caries-preventive measure; that is, tooth movement may relieve crowding or other conditions that hinder oral hygiene efforts. However, all orthodontic therapy represents a serious invasion of the oral environment. The numerous orthodontic components encourage the accumulation of plaque and the proliferation of bacteria, increasing the risk of caries and periodontitis. Orthodontists are all too familiar with the oral health problems that may be initiated by fixed appliances: massive initial lesions and even more advanced enamel loss following the removal of wires and brackets.

A sensible approach to the avoidance of such conditions is a systematic program for prevention of caries and periodontal diseases. Orthodontists are responsible for helping their patients to achieve adequate oral hygiene and for identifying and guiding patients with poor oral hygiene. Patients, and in the case of the young, parents, often do not take responsibility for their oral health and are indifferent to oral health-care measures. Because caries and periodontitis are rarely life threatening, these conditions are commonly ignored. Effective preventive oral health care is needed and should consist of education of the patient (and parent) and early diagnosis of dental and periodontal diseases. In the event of poor compliance with treatment, the orthodontist must have the courage to discontinue treatment.

Rarely in medicine is the relationship between a disease and its prevention so clear and scientifically documented as in the etiology of caries and periodontitis. This book explains the etiology of caries and periodontitis and the methods available for evaluating the patient's risk of experiencing these conditions. Subsequent chapters discuss means of minimizing the orthodontic patient's risk of caries and periodontitis through professional and at-home reduction of oral bacteria. The book's final chapter presents a systematic program for preventing oral health problems in orthodontic patients. This comprehensive analysis of the factors involved in the development and prevention of caries and periodontitis will provide clinicians with the means to develop individualized preventive programs for patients with orthodontic appliances.

The aforementioned increase in the number of patients who wear orthodontic appliances makes this book a must for general dentists and periodontists who treat orthodontic patients as well as for orthodontists who wish to establish a truly preventive approach to treatment.

Effects of Orthodontic Treatment on Oral Health

PURPORTED BENEFITS OF ORTHODONTIC TREATMENT

Proponents of classic orthodontics have always sought to define biological-medical indications for treatment. The elimination and prevention of dysfunctional disturbances in the stomatognathic system and the prevention of caries and periodontal disease have been the chief motivators. In addition, orthodontic treatment can correct orofacial conditions that deviate from existing social standards. Such conditions may influence the patient's psyche and integration in the social environment. However, the correlation between malocclusion and dysfunctions of any sort has been questioned in the more recent dental literature. Thus, it appears reasonable to evaluate the clinical claims of the benefits of orthodontic treatment. After all, absent some benefit, no medical indication for any sort of intervention exists.

Prevention of orofacial disturbances

According to traditional orthodontic theory, deviations of the tooth position and skeletal relationship can cause disturbances of the occlusion and the temporomandibular joint, as well as disturbances of

growth of the face and the dentition. Available scientific studies are not sufficient, however, to prove such claims. For example, there is no statistically significant correlation between occlusal disturbances of various types and mandibular dysfunction (Mohlin and Thilander 1984). However, in the individual patient, orthodontic treatment can worsen or even elicit existing disturbances of the temporomandibular joint.

Nevertheless, orthodontic therapy can be beneficial in patients with certain specific conditions. The mere existence of one of these types of malposition is not an absolute indication for orthodontic therapy, but studies have suggested that:

1. Correction of protruding maxillary anterior teeth reduces the risk of tooth trauma in the event of an accident (Jarvinen 1979).

2. Extensive flaring of the maxillary anterior teeth is a cofactor for drifting of these teeth in adulthood.

3. Impacted teeth can lead to pathologic consequences, including impeded eruption of adjacent teeth, root resorption of adjacent teeth, increased risk of fracture of the mandible, and cystic or malignant degeneration (Bishara and Andreasen 1983).

4. An impinging overbite may be associated with traumatization of the palatal and buccal mucosa.

Prevention of caries and periodontitis

Unfavorable anatomic conditions, particularly crowding, can increase the risk of caries because plaque retention is elevated, in part because the patient has greater difficulty in maintaining oral hygiene (Miller and Hobson 1961, Katz 1977). Orthodontic treatment can provide relief in such instances (Figs 1-1; 1-2a and 1-2b).

Nevertheless, no correlation was found between positional anomalies and caries prevalence in a 20-year longitudinal study of patients with various anomalies (crossbite, excessive overjet, or crowding) and a control group (Helm and Petersen 1989a). With respect to periodontal conditions, a small statistically significant difference was found between the groups, but only when excessive overjet, crossbite, or crowding was present (Helm and Petersen 1989b). Periodontal conditions were registered applying the CPITN-index

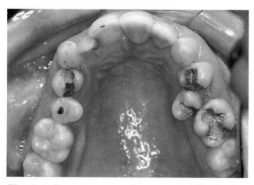

Fig 1-1 Extreme crowding, especially in the maxillary premolar region, made the less-than-optimal oral hygiene more difficult and thus supported development of caries in the now restored teeth.

(sound, calculus, gingivitis, pocket 3–5 mm, pocket >5 mm). These studies demonstrated that neither caries prevention nor preventive periodontics alone justifies orthodontic elimination of positional anomalies of the teeth and jaws. To express the authors' conclusions in another way, specific professional oral hygiene techniques are just as dependable as orthodontic therapy for preventing destruction of dental hard tissue and the tooth-supporting apparatus.

The relationship between tooth malpositioning, crowding in particular, and caries is controversial (Fig 1-3). Furthermore, there has been some discussion of whether, and to what extent, positional anomalies (severe crowding in particular) and the development of gingivitis and periodontitis can be associated. Although some correlation has been found between crowding and the accumulation of plaque or the degree of gingivitis (Ainamo 1972, Silness and Roynstrand 1985), other authors have reached the opposite conclusion (Geiger et al 1974, Ingervall et al 1977, Buckley 1981). However, this apparent contradiction can be explained by the differences in the study groups (patient age and, more importantly, oral hygiene status). Furthermore, the definition of crowding varied among the studies.

Ingervall and coworkers (1977), in their 6-month study of 50 21- to 32-year-old patients, concluded that the determining factor for gingival inflammation is more likely the amount of the accumulated plaque than the crowding itself. When cleaning of the interdental spaces was stopped, plaque accumulation and symptoms of gingivitis resulted on teeth in normal position as well as the crowded teeth. When the subjects resumed regular use of dental floss, the plaque and gingival index scores decreased similarly in both groups.

This finding was confirmed in a more recent study by Davies and coworkers (1991). Although the orthodontically treated patients had lower plaque and gingival index scores than the untreated control group after 3 years, the difference was ascribed more to greater awareness of oral hygiene than to the orthodontic therapy itself. Thus, it can be concluded that malaligned teeth contribute to the establishment of periodontal disease only when oral hygiene is poor or average.

In certain instances, however, orthodontic measures have an indisputably positive effect on the periodontium when anomalies of tooth position are accompanied by chronic traumatic contact of the oral mucosa by teeth (Poulton 1989).

Although still controversial, preprosthetic uprighting of tipped mandibular molars is said to lead to an improvement in periodontal conditions (Lang 1977) (Figs 1-4a and 1-4b). Similarly, intrusion of teeth with severe periodontal damage can lead to formation of new attachment if oral hygiene is perfect and periodontal therapy is provided at the initiation of and throughout the treatment period (Melsen et al 1988, 1989). In general, however, presumably there is no scientific proof that orthodontic therapy alone has a positive effect on the health of, or the restoration of health to, tooth-supporting soft tissue or dental hard tissue. Orthodontic measures may help to simplify plaque removal and thus contribute to more effective oral hygiene.

Improvement of esthetics and psychosocial well-being

The external appearance of an individual influences interpersonal relationships to an extent that should not be underestimated. Teachers, for example, anticipate that unattractive students will attain lower levels of

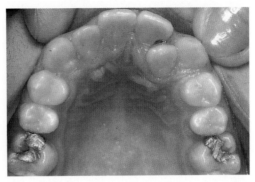

Fig 1-2a Crowding can lead to excessive plaque accumulation and subsequent caries, as on the distal surface of the maxillary left central incisor. Even in the presence of extreme crowding, tooth destruction can be impeded by thorough interdental care.

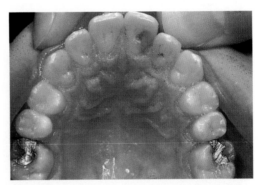

Fig 1-2b Same patient as in Fig 1-2a after orthodontic therapy and temporary restoration.

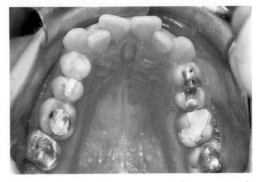

Fig 1-3 Despite extreme crowding, no proximal caries has developed in the maxillary anterior teeth of this patient because of his good oral hygiene practices.

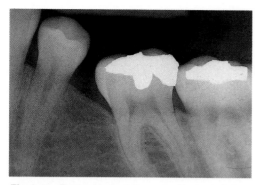

Fig 1-4a Radiograph of the mandibular left first molar before treatment.

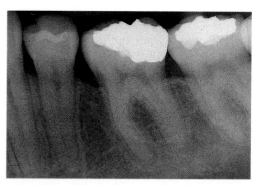

Fig 1-4b Radiograph of the same tooth after 2 years of orthodontic therapy. Note the increase in attachment.

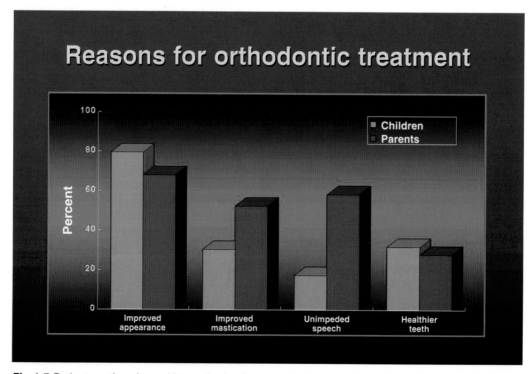

Fig 1-5 Patient motives in seeking orthodontic treatment.

education and academic achievement (Clifford 1975). If the appeal of the child is judged solely by his or her dental appearance, it has only a minor effect on the teacher's expectations (Shaw and Humphreys 1982). Nonetheless, 70% of parents questioned expressed the belief that orthodontic therapy made their children more attractive, and 75% believed that it would contribute to the later career success of the child (Shaw et al 1979).

An unattractive child may be teased by his or her playmates, which may cause life-long trauma (Helm et al 1985). Adults may be disadvantaged in the search for a mate and in finding suitable employment. Potential consequences of these experiences include the development of inferiority or other psychological complexes (Helm et al 1985).

Thus, the contribution of orthodontics to the health of the entire stomatognathic system should not be overvalued. The indications for therapy arise not so much from medical-biologic grounds as they do from psychological or simply esthetic reasons (Fig 1-5).

RISKS OF ORTHODONTIC TREATMENT

Orthodontic movement of teeth can elicit alterations in the tooth-supporting apparatus and in dental hard tissues. Most common among these are root resorption, gingival recession, and an increased risk of caries and periodontitis.

Root resorption

It has been known for some time that root resorption, predominantly of the root tip, can be a consequence of orthodontic therapy (Fig 1-6). Although the lateral portions of the root are sometimes partially resorbed, such processes, unlike apical resorptions, are frequently repaired through the deposition of osteocementum.

In general, the cause of and the mechanism underlying such degenerative processes remain undefined. Because root resorption is also found in patients who have never had orthodontic treatment, a direct cause-and-effect relationship between tooth movement and root resorption is questionable (Vanarsdall 1991).

Resorption is an unpredictable event. Empirical data permit some conclusions about patients who may be at risk, however. They include:

1. Patients who already have some apical resorption on at least one tooth.
2. Patients with short or narrow roots.
3. Patients with anterior open bite.
4. Patients with traumatically injured anterior teeth.

Furthermore, resorption is more common in adults than in younger patients and is particularly common in the maxillary lateral incisors. The assumption that endodontically treated teeth are at greater risk for root resorption than vital teeth has been disproven (Spurrier et al 1990).

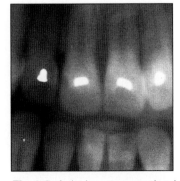

Fig 1-6 Apical root resorption in the maxillary anterior region in a patient treated for several years with fixed appliances.

Orthodontists should examine all available radiographs so that potential resorptions can be diagnosed at an early stage and the treatment plan can be altered as necessary.

Gingival recession

Dehiscence of the alveolar bone is a prerequisite for the development of gingival recession (Bernimoulin and Curiloviç 1977). Pronounced labial movement of the incisors, particularly in the form of tipping, favors the appearance of such dehiscences. If a tooth with bony dehiscence is guided lingually again, a new bone lamella forms (Thilander et al 1983).

Recessions occur less commonly when a thick attached gingiva is present. Not only the width but also the volume of the attached gingiva is decisive (Wennström et al 1987). Once established, recessions do not show a tendency to progress (Årtun and Krogstad 1987). Spontaneous resolution of recession occasionally arises in children after the eruption of the mandibular incisors (Andlin-Sobocki et al 1991).

Caries and periodontitis

Removable appliances

Removable orthodontic appliances include numerous different therapeutic devices, eg, active plates, retention plates, bite planes, stimulation plates, functional devices, and inclined planes. Each of these appliances consists of a resin body as well as retentive and active elements, usually fabricated of metal. The instructions for use of removable orthodontic appliances varies greatly. For example, stimulation plates are inserted several times daily for brief periods in cerebral palsy patients, but Fränkel appliances are worn almost constantly. The same is true for inclined planes, which must remain in the mouth even while the patient is eating.

In view of the numerous designs and the great variation in the amount of time that such appliances are worn, it is difficult to formulate generally effective rules for oral hygiene practices required of patients who use removable orthodontic appliances.

Patients who are being treated with removable appliances can practice oral hygiene in the usual manner. After removal of the appliance from the mouth, patients can use a toothbrush and dental floss just as do patients who are not being treated orthodontically.

That oral hygiene is simpler for children with removable appliances than it is for children with fixed appliances was confirmed by Schlagenhauf et al (1989). They found that the number of *Streptococcus mutans* does not increase significantly in patient who wear removable appliances, in contrast to findings in patients with fixed appliances. Nor does treatment with active plates or functional orthodontic appliances lead to periodontal disease in any other way (Flores de Jacoby and Müller 1982). However, it has been established that inflammation of the palatal gingiva occurs more frequently in patients wearing removable appliances than in those treated with fixed appliances (Pender 1986).

The greater accumulation of plaque on dental materials than on natural enamel must be considered (Skjörland 1973) (Figs 1-7a and 1-7b). Because of their microporosity, the surface of resins is coated quickly with streptococci in particular and with gram-positive and gram-negative rods and yeasts (Bickel and Geering 1982). This increase in microorganisms increases the risk of carious lesions and prosthetic stomatitis (Schröder 1982) (Fig 1-8).

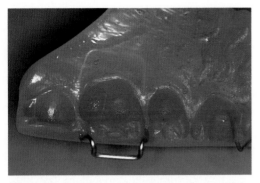

Fig 1-7a Activator with plaque disclosed to demonstrate that removable appliances contribute to the accumulation of plaque.

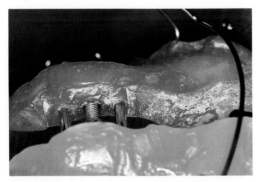

Fig 1-7b Activator with calculus as a sign of poor appliance hygiene and oral hygiene.

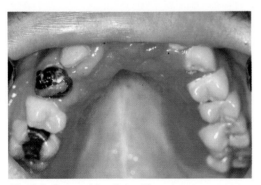

Fig 1-8 Stomatitis elicited by excess monomer in the resin of a removable orthodontic appliance; poor oral hygiene may have acted as a cofactor.

Fixed appliances

Injuries to dental hard tissue arising from fixed appliances are the result of technical-operative measures or changes in the environment of the oral cavity.

Abrasion and hard tissue defects. Placement of fixed appliances almost always leads to loss, directly or indirectly, of dental hard tissue. The process of bonding and debonding orthodontic devices removes 30 to 42 μm of enamel, through polishing of the tooth surface, the etching procedure, removal of excess resin composite with rotating instruments, and, in particular, removal of the brackets and the associated finishing of the enamel surface (Pus and Way 1980). An even greater loss occurs when filled resin composites are used. The loss of dental enamel is greatest (up to 72 μm) if a bracket loosens repeatedly and requires rebonding (Thompson and Way 1981).

Actual tearouts of enamel may occur during removal of ceramic brackets because of their great adhesion. For that reason, such brackets should be used only with strict attention to indication (esthetic requirements of the patient during the treatment phase) and only on selected teeth (ie, teeth with no visible surface alterations such as enamel cracks or initial carious lesions) (Ghafari 1992). To prevent enamel tearouts, thermal debonding, in which the adhesive resin is softened, was developed (Jost-Brinkmann et al 1989), Jost-Brinkmann et al 1992). To prevent such damage to enamel, numerous ceramic brackets today are manufactured not with a silanized, but rather with a mechanically retentive, base. Neither the defects described earlier nor enamel cracks occur with metal brackets if they are placed and removed in accordance with established procedures (Zachrisson et al

1980). A remaining problem of ceramic brackets relates to their hardness, which can lead to attrition of the opposing teeth (Viazis et al 1989).

Plaque accumulation. Although fixed orthodontic appliances have the advantage of three-dimensional control of tooth movement and therefore are used increasingly everywhere, they represent a special stress on the oral environment. Bands, brackets, arch wires, and other devices can easily upset the sensitive biologic balance of the oral cavity (Fig 1-9). The appliances allow increased plaque accumulation. Plaque accumulates particularly beneath bands from which some cement has been washed out (Mizrahi 1982), on composite surfaces adjacent to adhesive retention elements, and on interfaces between composite and enamel (Gwinnett and Ceen 1979) (Figs 1-10a and 1-10b). Plaque is found predominantly cervical to brackets and under arch wires (Fig 1-11).

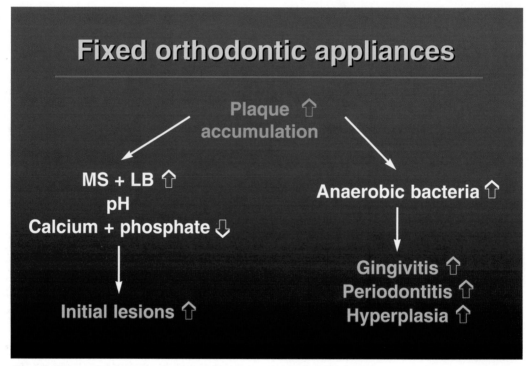

Fig 1-9 Effect of fixed orthodontic appliances on the oral environment.

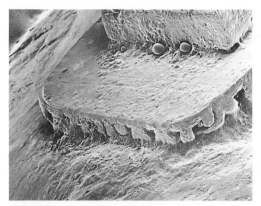

Fig 1-10a Scanning electron microscopic view of plaque at the metal-composite–enamel interface. (Original magnification x 44.)

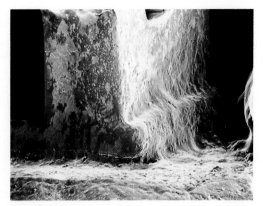

Fig 1-10b Scanning electron microscopic view of plaque on the bracket itself. (Original magnification x 44.)

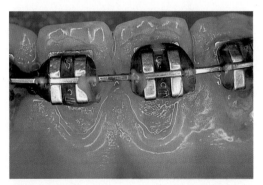

Fig 1-11 Mandibular incisors with brackets. Stained plaque is present especially in the proximal and cervical regions.

Demineralization. Beneath such plaque, superficial enamel may quickly be demineralized (O'Reilly and Featherstone 1987). Consequently, white spot lesions can be observed at these plaque retention sites (Ceen and Gwinnett 1981, Øgaard et al 1988a). According to Gorelick and coworkers (1982), the appearance and distribution of sites of demineralization are highly variable. In general, demineralization occurs in the anterior maxillary teeth and in the posterior teeth of the mandible (Figs 1-12a and 1-12b). One explanation for this pronounced distribution pattern is that these tooth surfaces lie beyond the re-

gions controlled by saliva next to the salivary ducts. A comparison between a treatment group and a control group that was not treated orthodontically showed that the treatment group had approximately three times as high a risk of demineralization, calculated for individual teeth. On the whole, however, the incidence of demineralization was slight (Gorelick et al 1982). White spots with established cavitation were found in only seven patients.

A later study found a correlation between the duration of treatment and the appearance of minor and deep demineralization (Geiger et al 1988). The probability of a lesion was higher in patients who wore fixed appliances for more than 2 years. In addition to teeth with brackets, 280 banded maxillary anterior teeth were examined; of these, 12% showed white spots when the bands were removed.

Such demineralization, however, is not so much a consequence of an increased volume of plaque, but rather the result of a simultaneously occurring differentiation to an especially cariogenic microflora that increases the risk of caries. Specifically, the differentiation of the microflora leads to a greater concentration of

9

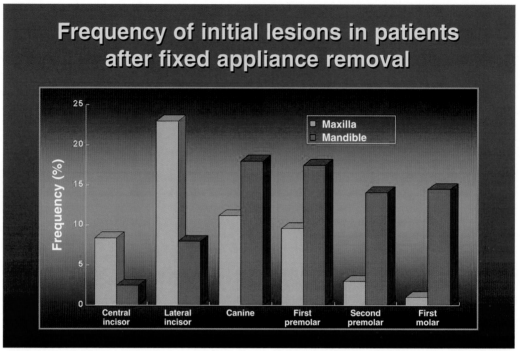

Fig 1-12a Redrawn from Gorelick et al 1982.

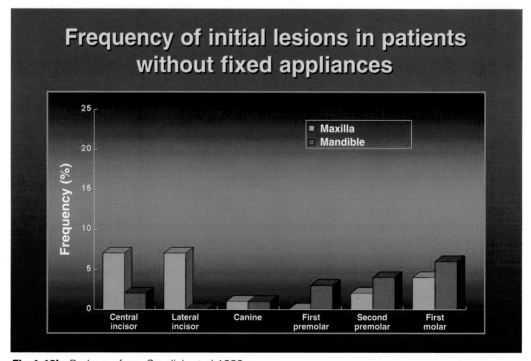

Fig 1-12b Redrawn from Gorelick et al 1982.

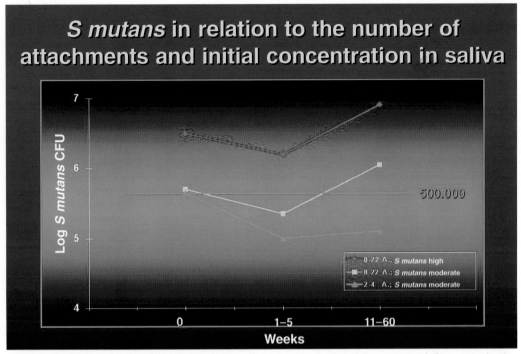

Fig 1-13 Relationship between the number of attachments and the amount of *S mutans* in the saliva. (Redrawn from Scheie et al 1984.)

acid-forming bacteria while extracellular and intracellular polysaccharides increase (Balenseifen and Madonia 1970). At the same time, the free calcium and phosphate ions that are required for remineralization decrease in concentration (Chatterjee and Kleinberg 1979).

Bacterial proliferation. *Streptococcus mutans* and lactobacilli are among the acid-forming microorganisms that proliferate. Fixed appliances and brackets provide ideal conditions for growth of the latter, because lactobacilli multiply on every retention surface, in every carious pit, just as they do on bands and brackets (Sakamaki and Bahn 1968). The same is true of *S mutans,* though to a lesser degree (Corbett et al 1981, Mattingly et al 1983, Scheie et al 1984, Rosenbloom and Tinanoff 1991). These bacteria are among the principal causational agents of caries.

A study by Corbett et al (1981) showed that caries-free banded patients have far more *S mutans* in their plaque (buccolingual and proximal) than do nonbanded subjects. Scheie and coworkers (1984) observed an initial reduction in *S mutans* in plaque and saliva, which they ascribed to destruction of the bacterial reservoir during the banding process. After 3 months, however, the density of *S mutans* organisms in saliva and plaque far exceeded initial values. In contrast, nonbanded teeth experienced only a slight increase in *S mutans.* Furthermore, it was shown simultaneously that the amount of *S mutans* in the saliva increased almost exponentially with the number of bands and brackets (Fig 1-13). The enhanced local growth increased the level of infection; the number of organisms in plaque taken from nonbanded adjacent teeth also increased in patients who had more than eight bands and brackets.

Rosenbloom and Tinanoff (1991) compared *S mutans* values of saliva of patients in the active orthodontic treatment phase with those of subjects in retention, subjects who were postretention, and a control group with no orthodontic devices of any sort. Only those patients wearing fixed appliances had increased *S mutans* levels. All other subjects, including those wearing fixed or removable retainers, demonstrated only small numbers of *S mutans*. The authors concluded that no long-lasting increase in *S mutans* levels needs to be anticipated solely on the basis of the wearing of fixed orthodontic appliances.

Over the average 2-year treatment period, however, cariogenic bacteria, and the mutans streptococci group in particular, have sufficient time to form carious lesions. On average, 1 year is required for a carious lesion to become established, and 3 years are needed for it to reach the dentin (Berman and Slack 1973, Newbrun 1989). It may be assumed that, in the presence of increased numbers of *S mutans* and the corresponding retention surfaces, the carious process is significantly accelerated.

Because *S mutans* colonizes particularly well in the proximal spaces of the mo-

lars, which are poorly accessible to oral hygiene, these regions, together with the occlusal surfaces, are particularly prone to carious attack (Kristoffersson et al 1984). Thus, bands and brackets significantly increase the risk to the already endangered molars. A related study (Schlagenhauf et al 1989) compared the effects of fixed and removable appliance therapy on the bacterial flora and demonstrated that the *S mutans* count was clearly elevated only in patients with fixed appliances.

Caries. The inescapable consequence of increased *S mutans* values would be, in principle, an increase in the incidence of caries, because that organism is held to be the most important bacterium for the initiation of caries. In patients with fixed orthodontic appliances, the proximal spaces and the smooth surfaces around brackets are exposed to the greatest risk for caries (Gorelick et al 1982) (Figs 1-14a and 1-14b). If a massive excess of resin composite that may extend into the proximal region remains after brackets are bonded, plaque retention is increased enormously (Fig 1-15).

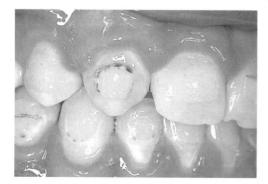 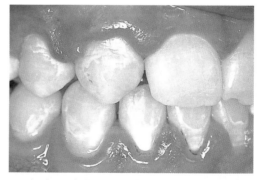

Figs 1-14a and 1-14b Photograph taken at the conclusion of fixed appliance therapy. Demineralization, the extent of which becomes clearly apparent only after all adhesive remnants have been removed, has occurred around numerous brackets.

Zachrisson and Zachrisson (1971) investigated the increase in the number of caries lesions in fully banded patients who had been treated an average of 19 months. To ensure correct diagnosis of caries, bitewing radiographs were taken before and after the completion of therapy. Surprisingly, the results showed no great increase in the incidence of caries in fully banded patients; rather, a shift in location of caries from proximal to buccal and lingual sites was found. Teeth on which attachments had been placed buccally or lingually had higher rates of caries. The investigators concluded that bands that surround the entire tooth contribute to caries protection. Similar results were reported by Ingervall (1962).

Most problems arise only when bands loosen or form shoulders (Corbett et al 1981). The fact that bands are rarely adapted exactly to the tooth surface also is a disadvantage; sites always exist where the band is not in close contact with the tooth and where the cement layer is relatively thick (Fig 1-16).

In principle, every treatment with fixed appliances increases the risk of caries significantly. In practice, that means that bands do not automatically provide better caries protection than brackets. Tooth surfaces with properly placed bands are, indeed, protected temporarily, but the cement used to fix the bands can be washed out. The cement loss results in a micro-gap in which caries can become established almost without being disturbed (Fig 1-17). Similarly, if the bracket adhesive does not cover a bracket base completely, a carious lesion can develop quickly, without being noticed, in any gap that exists (Figs 1-18a and 1-18b; 1-19).

Caries also can arise immediately adjacent to orthodontic bands. The gingival margin is a region deserving increased

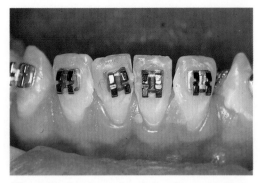

Fig 1-15 Brackets bonded with an indirect technique with significant excess composite. This type of excess leads to increased plaque retention and, thereby, increased risk of caries.

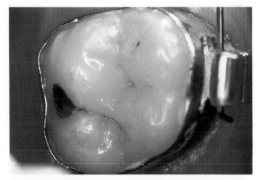

Fig 1-16 Because the margins of orthodontic bands almost never fit the tooth surface perfectly, the marginal regions are always potential spaces for plaque accumulation.

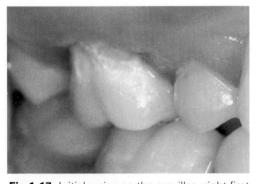

Fig 1-17 Initial caries on the maxillary right first molar after removal of a band. In addition, numerous signs of demineralization indicate poor oral hygiene.

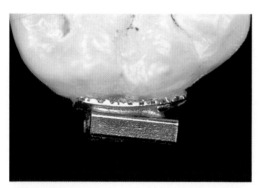

Fig 1-18a Retention niche for cariogenic plaque bacteria formed at a site that is difficult to observe clinically and therefore prone to (secondary) caries.

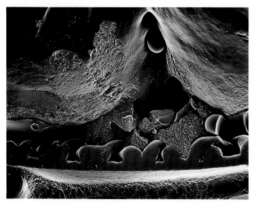

Fig 1-18b Scanning electron microscopic view of the same tooth as in Fig 1-18a. (Original magnification x 36.)

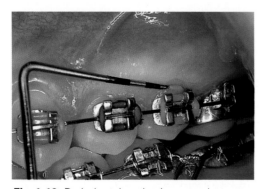

Fig 1-19 Periodontal probe in a gap between the enamel surface and an unacceptable, dangerous composite resin excess.

attention. For reasons of caries prevention, therefore, many respected clinicians recommend that band margins not be placed subgingivally. If this situation cannot be avoided, despite reduction of the width of the band, a gingivectomy is recommended (Anderman 1989).

Gingivitis and periodontitis. Subgingival crown and restoration margins always are associated with inflammation of the adjacent connective tissue (Renggli 1974). This type of inflammation has also been demonstrated with orthodontic bands (Zachrisson and Zachrisson 1972, Zachrisson 1976, Legott et al 1984, Huser et al 1990), and may result in loss of attachment (Zachrisson and Alnæs 1973) (Figs 1-20 and 1-21). Boyd and Baumrind (1992) found that all measured parameters (plaque index, gingival index, bleeding index, and probing depth) were higher for banded molars than for molars with brackets. The loss of attachment was highest proximally, particularly in adults. The margins of bands usually were subgingival proximally.

Bands with subgingival margins also displace plaque subgingivally and thereby foster gingivitis or even periodontitis (Ericsson et al 1977). As is the case in overhanging restoration margins, gram-negative anaerobic organisms, such as *Porphyromonas gingivalis* (formerly *Bacteroides gingivalis*) as well as *Prevotella intermedia* (formerly *Bacteroides intermedius*) and *Actinomyces* species, are disproportionately present along the subgingival band margins (Diamanti-Kipioti et al 1987).

Gingival inflammation in the presence of orthodontic bands also may be associated with increased numbers of spirochetes, mobile rods, and fusiform organisms, and a simultaneous decrease in the

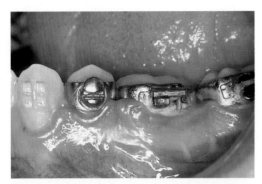

Fig 1-20 Subgingivally located band. Severe plaque accumulation has caused development of periodontal disease.

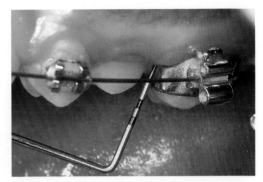

Fig 1-21 Subgingival band with signs of inflammation of the marginal gingiva. Probing depth is 3 mm.

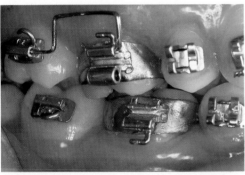

Fig 1-22 Orthodontic bands on the first molars after appropriate reduction of the gingival margin buccally (and lingually). The interproximal region remains a problem.

proportion of cocci (Müller and Flores de Jacoby 1982, Huser et al 1990). The condition of the gingiva worsens during orthodontic treatment with fixed appliances, even when personal oral hygiene practices are good (Hartmann et al 1982). Only the removal of bands and brackets, together with continuing good oral hygiene, can lead to a complete resolution of gingivitis (Atherton 1970). Without professional plaque removal, however, persistent changes in the subgingival flora can be found on teeth that had carried bands or brackets, even years after completion of

orthodontic treatment (Freundorfer et al 1993). Freundorfer et al (1993) also reported that teeth that had been banded always had a greater proportion of spirochetes than did those to which brackets had been bonded.

Because many clinicians do not take the time to refine bands so that their margins lie supragingivally, bonding of brackets by the acid-etch technique is always preferable to cementation of bands (Fig 1-22). A prospective long-term study by Miethke and Bernimoulin (1988) showed that, except for the plaque index, all measures of the periodontal condition of banded teeth were significantly ($p < 0.5$) worse 1 year after placement than were those of teeth on which brackets had been placed (Figs 1-23a to 1-23c). For gingival health, therefore, brackets are more favorable, provided that excess adhesive is removed carefully (Fig 1-24).

Contribution of dental materials. It is well accepted that various dental materials accumulate more plaque than does dental enamel; this is true for steel bands, adhesive cements (Ørstavik and Ørstavik 1981), and resin composite materials

Figs 1-23a to 1-23c Distribution of microbes in the plaque of three groups of teeth after 1 year of orthodontic treatment. The teeth were fitted alternately with bands and brackets, with a crossover design between both sides and jaws so that an intraindividual comparison was possible. (From Miethke and Bernimoulin 1988.)

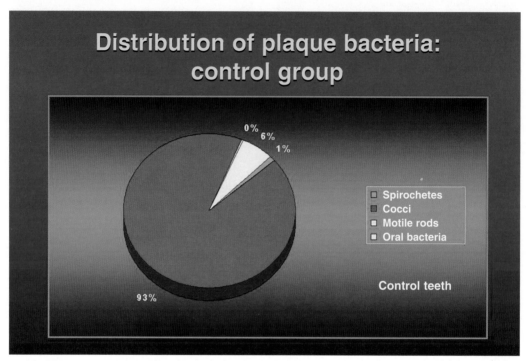

Fig 1-23a

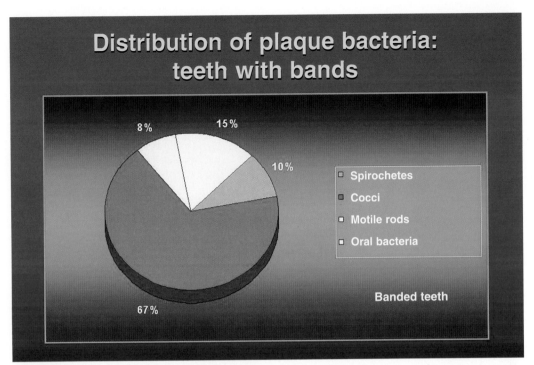

Fig 1-23b

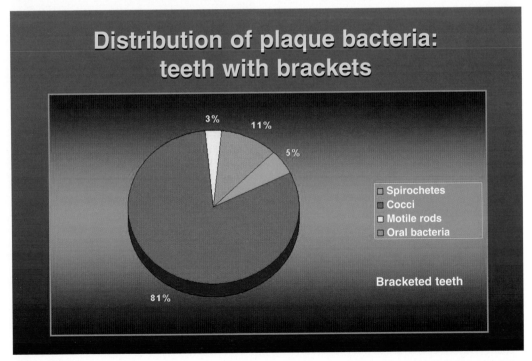

Fig 1-23c

(Skjörland 1973). Besides the surface characteristics of dental materials, other factors also determine plaque accumulation. All surfaces exposed in the oral cavity rapidly absorb salivary proteins, thereby changing the physicochemical properties of the material and the interaction between material, pellicle, and bacteria (Ørstavik 1980). Excess composite adhesive can lead rapidly to inflammation, particularly in the interdental region (Zachrisson and Brobakken 1976).

Obviously, aging of the material plays a role in plaque formation and retention. Van Dijken and colleagues (1987) found no differences in plaque and gingivitis indices between natural dental enamel and subgingival composite restorations, regardless of the type of composite used (conventional, hybrid, or microfilled), 1 year after placement of the restorations. However, the difference between natural enamel and composite restorations became significant after 2 years.

The clinician can attempt to reduce the problem of secondary caries associated with banding by adding fluoride (Shannon 1981, Hastreiter 1989) or, as is becoming more common, by using glass-ionomer cement, which releases fluoride ions (Forss and Seppä 1990, Forsten 1990). A study by Svanberg and coworkers (1990) demonstrated that *S mutans* is less prevalent on glass-ionomer cement than on composite or amalgam restorations. An in vitro study revealed that bands fixed with glass-ionomer cement elicit less mineral loss than do those cemented with materials that do not release fluoride (Rezk-Lega et al 1991).

Copper cements also are used for band cementation (Jost-Brinkmann et al 1989). Copper cements are zinc phosphate cements to which various types of copper compounds have been added so that the antimicrobial properties of metallic

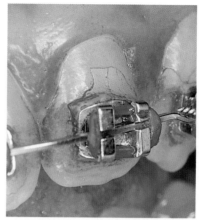

Fig 1-24 Excess adhesive with accumulated plaque around the brackets on the lateral incisor and canine. Plaque is disclosed by malachite green.

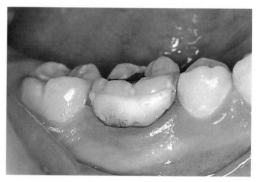

Fig 1-25 Mandibular right first molar after loss of a band that had been fixed with glass-ionomer cement. The cement adheres primarily to the enamel and thereby prevents demineralization.

copper can hinder the development of caries. Although the bactericidal properties of copper cements have been confirmed in vitro (Finster and Riethe 1963), their effectiveness in vivo has yet to be demonstrated and must be doubted on the basis of recent findings (Jost-Brinkmann et al 1994).

Regardless of the cement used, the problem of cement washout remains, although glass-ionomer cement is said to be clearly less soluble than zinc phosphate cement (Maijer and Smith 1988). When bands fixed with glass-ionomer cement loosen, the weak point lies at the cement–band interface. The cement remains protectively on the tooth surface (Norris et al 1986) (Fig 1-25). Nevertheless, every type of luting of bands and brackets increases plaque retention. More plaque, in turn, harbors more cariogenic bacteria. Where more *S mutans* exist, more caries may be anticipated (Kristoffersson et al 1985).

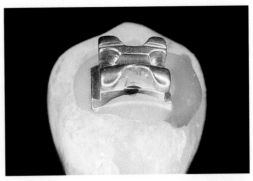

Fig 1-26 Extracted premolar to which a bracket had been bonded. The pink region depicts an unetched area that had been covered by adhesive resin. Erythrosin has entered the gap. In vivo the possibility of inflow would exist for nearly all microorganisms.

PREVENTION OF ORAL HEALTH PROBLEMS

In addition to the use of fluorides, Zachrisson (1977) recommended that the composite or sealant used to bond brackets be extended to the gingival margin, to prevent demineralization of the cervical regions of the enamel surface. This suggestion is problematic, however, because almost all sealants have a degree of cytotoxicity. Furthermore, polymerization does not take place outside the bracket base in pressure-polymerizing adhesives (Tell et al 1988). The best composite–enamel adaptation with a smooth composite surface is achieved, according to scanning microscopic studies, when an unfilled bonding agent is used, the brackets are coated optimally with composite, and the excess is not removed with an instrument (Oliver and Howe 1989).

This last bit of advice must be considered carefully, however. Is it not specifically the excess materials that accelerate plaque accumulation and thus may cause problems such as demineralization? All types of gingival irritation should be avoided. The use of small bracket bases and the careful removal of excess adhesive contribute to the relative maintenance of gingival health. Only minor gingival inflammation occurs at bracket sites when good oral hygiene is practiced (Zachrisson and Zachrisson 1972). Similarly, composite remnants on unetched enamel can act like fine marginal gaps on restorations that lead quickly to demineralization and "secondary caries" under the composite (Fig 1-26).

Because orthodontic therapy, particularly with fixed appliances, increases the risk of caries, conscientious efforts on the part of the dentist and the patient are mandatory. The emphasis on strict oral hygiene practices during orthodontic therapy may instill long-term "prevention consciousness" in patients. Good prevention-oriented attitudes can be set, as has been demonstrated in controlled studies. Feliu (1982) compared the oral hygiene of 74 orthodontically treated patients with that of 74 untreated subjects and found that the gingivitis and plaque indices of the treated subjects were lower than those of the untreated individuals. Southard and coworkers (1986) found that caries prevalence was lower in orthodontically treated naval recruits than in an untreated group. The finding was related to better education in caries prevention during orthodontic therapy.

Orthodontic patients need not even fear a greater risk of periodontal disease, as long as orthodontic therapy is accompanied by an adequate program of prophylaxis (Huber et al 1987, Lervik and Haugejorden 1988).

Even patients with advanced periodontal disease can be treated successfully (Figs 1-27a to 1-27g), provided that systematic periodontal therapy leading to inflammation-free periodontal tissue is given beforehand and that this condition is maintained during orthodontic therapy. Development of periodontal lesions essentially is impossible if consistent plaque control exists, because the young dentition is less susceptible (Zachrisson and Alnæs 1973, Alstad and Zachrisson 1979).

In contrast, gingival hyperplasia poses a significant problem. Gingival hyperplasia is found almost routinely with the lingual technique but occurs to an irregular extent even with labially attached brackets. In a longitudinal study, Zachrisson and Zachrisson (1972) found moderate gingival hyperplasia on nearly all teeth of many of 49 subjects treated with fixed appliances. Hyperplasia may occur to an even greater extent and can be generalized. Gingival hyperplasia complicates oral hygiene significantly; any manipulation in the patient's mouth, eg, cementing of bands or brackets, is impeded. Despite frequent professional cleaning of the teeth, hyperplastic tissue sometimes persists and must be removed surgically (Figs 1-28a and 1-28b). Recurrences are frequent especially if a high standard of professional hygiene is not ensured.

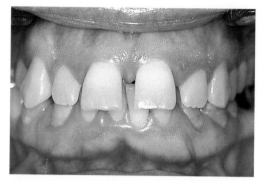

Fig 1-27a Adult patient with advanced periodontitis before orthodontic therapy.

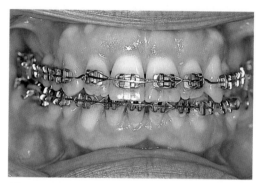

Fig 1-27b Same patient during orthodontic therapy.

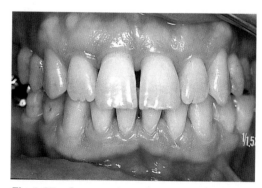

Fig 1-27c Same patient after orthodontic therapy.

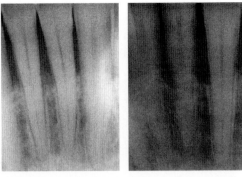 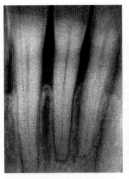 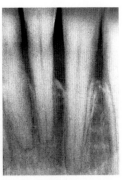

Fig 1-27d Periodontal condition of the anterior region of the mandible before initiation of treatment.

Fig 1-27e Although the overall periodontal condition has not worsened, slight apical resorption is apparent at the conclusion of treatment.

Figs 1-27f and 1-27g Periodontal conditions before and after orthodontic correction. (Periodontal treatment by S. Hägewald.)

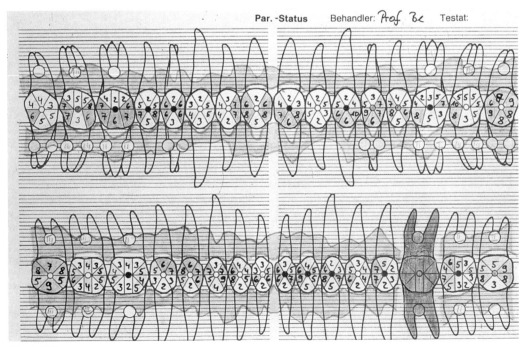

Fig 1-27f

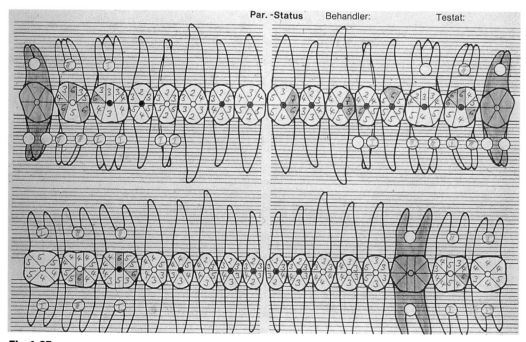

Fig 1-27g

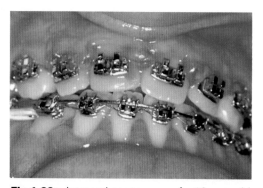

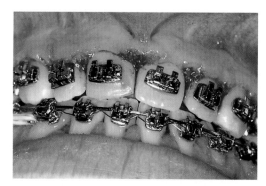

Fig 1-28a Intraoral appearance of a 10-year-old girl during orthodontic therapy. Gingival hyperplasia, particularly in the maxillary anterior region, is an expression of poor oral hygiene.

Fig 1-28b Same patient following gingivectomy in the maxillary anterior region.

CONCLUSIONS

Orthodontic treatment by itself rarely has a preventive effect on caries or periodontal disease, but it can help to simplify oral hygiene and thus make it more effective. Orthodontic therapy with removable appliances causes no significant additional problems for the oral environment. However, the fixed installation of retentive elements that remain in the mouth for at least 1 or 2 years results in a multiplication of cariogenic microorganisms. Similarly, an increase in gram-negative flora with a periodontal pathologic stimulus can be anticipated. The tendency to use brackets instead of bands more frequently has led to only a minor alleviation of the problem. Specific measures, therefore, are necessary to prevent damage that otherwise would occur almost automatically.

Evaluation of Oral Health and Measurement of Risk

2

P revention in orthodontics actually begins with the timely recognition and, if indicated, the prevention of tooth and jaw malpositioning, so that significant and long-lasting orthodontic therapy, which is associated with increased risk of caries, can be avoided or at least minimized. Because orthodontic anomalies usually are not the consequence of pathological processes but rather are disturbances in normal development, genetic and environmental factors act together in most orthodontic problems (Nakata and Wei 1988). During a child's active growth phase, dentofacial structures are significantly adaptable. Regular evaluation by the dentist or the orthodontist is necessary to establish the best time for initiation of treatment, so that the permanent teeth will erupt in their optimal positions. If therapy can be initiated at the right time, the orthodontist can make optimal use of physiologic growth and achieve the best possible alteration in the pattern of neuromuscular function.

In this manner, orthodontic treatment measures in children and adults could become simpler and shorter. (McNamara Jr and Brudon 1993) (Figs 2-1; 2-2a and 2-2b). At the same time, the dentist is challenged to explain to parents how preventive measures provide appro-priate conditions for comprehensive oral health. Because the average patient sees the dentist twice (or at best four times) annually, the child spends only 2 hours at the dentist's office. In those 2 hours, the dentist must do as much as possible to prevent oral health problems and motivate the patient to participate in prevention measures.

When comparing epidemiological data of two surveys from 1979–80 and 1988–91 for the United States, a significant caries decline has been observed for the 5- to 17-year-olds (Kaste et al 1996; NIDR 1982): the average number of carious or restored tooth surfaces was 2.5 in the late 1980s compared to 4.8 in the late 1970s. Furthermore, it is remarkable that in 1988–91 nearly 55% of the children of this age group had neither a restoration nor caries, whereas this number was 37% in the 1970s. If carious lesions were present, they were smaller in the 1980s than in the 1970s. Two thirds of these lesions were restricted to fissures and pits.

Caries decline is mostly attributed to the use of fluorides, especially fluoridated toothpaste and fluoridated water, but also to a higher tooth awareness, and alterations concerning diet may have contributed to the decline (Fejerskov 1995). In US adults, however, caries prevalence is still high. The mean number of decayed or

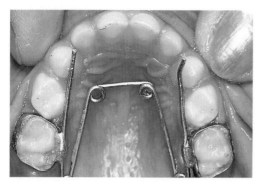

Fig 2-1 Early treatment of a crossbite using a Quadhelix in a primary dentition.

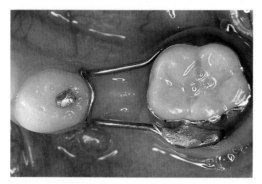

Fig 2-2a A spacer is used for extracted teeth. An orthodontic bond with a soldered arch is used for sagittal support.

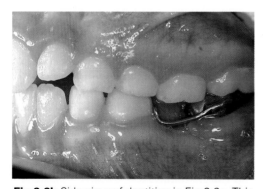

Fig 2-2b Side view of dentition in Fig 2-2a. This type of spacer is well suited to hold open the space for the coming permanent tooth. The way the supporting wire is positioned near the gingiva means it will not be bent out of shape by occlusal forces; however, the unsupported tooth may continue to grow.

restored coronal tooth surfaces was 21.5; caries was present in 94% of the 18- to 74-year-olds (Winn et al 1996); 22.5% of the dentate population was affected by root caries. Non-Hispanic blacks and Mexican Americans had significantly fewer carious lesions than non-Hispanic whites. Still, adults lose more teeth due to caries than to periodontitis (Phipps and Stevens 1995).

DIAGNOSIS OF CARIES

Fundamental to every step in dentistry is a comprehensive diagnosis of the problem, even in its earliest stages. For example, diagnosis of caries and the decisions for treatment arising from the diagnosis recently have reached a new standard. "Digging around" in initial carious lesions and in fissures is contraindicated, because the probe itself can carry caries-inducing microbes, and it is possible by probing to break through a still intact enamel layer, thus preventing remineralization (Bergman and Lindén 1969). That would provide the prerequisite conditions for the progression of isolated carious lesions (Ekstrand et al 1987).

Fissure caries

Clinical inspection can provide a relatively precise diagnosis for shallow V- and U-shaped fissures; diagnosis is much more difficult for deep, undercut, or bulb-shaped fissures. The first step in visual inspection is searching for zones of white demineralization around the entrance to the fissure. Such spots indicate the existence of undermining caries (Fig 2-3). Dark discoloration of a fissure indicates that the progress of caries has stopped. Downer (1975) found a strong correlation between

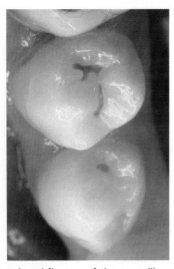

Fig 2-3 The discolored fissure of the mandibular second premolar has been irreversibly damaged by caries. The light color of the carious process indicates active caries. The whitish margins indicate the presence of an undermining process.

3. Transillumination of the occlusal region from the cervical aspect provides sound information for the experienced dentist (Pienihäkkinen 1990).

4. Softened carious dentin has less electrical resistance than sound dentin. A device is used to measure this difference. In comparative studies with histologic follow-up, this procedure had the highest accuracy (Verdonschot et al 1992). Reproducibility of the technique is higher than that of other procedures.

5. Recently, a new method, quantitative fluorescence radiography, showed promising results in the detection of occlusal caries of extracted teeth (Angmar-Månsson et al 1996). This method is, obviously, also highly precise in monitoring initial carious lesions that undergo intensive prophylactic care, as has been shown clinically in orthodontic patients (Angmar-Månsson et al 1996).

clinical visual diagnosis and histologic alterations.

Other procedures in establishing the diagnosis of fissure caries are:

1. The fissure may be explored with a (sharp) probe. "Sticking" of the probe at the entry funnel is not, however, a sure sign of fissure caries. A probe can "catch" on the narrow entrance of a fissure and appear to indicate softened dental hard tissue. Also problematic, as already noted, is the possible disturbance of an existing remineralization process.

2. Radiographs may be useful, but, as a rule, only relatively advanced lesions are recognizable on bitewing radiographs.

Proximal caries

Bitewing radiographs have special significance in the diagnosis of proximal caries (Figs 2-4a and 2-4b). However, in view of present knowledge about the possibilities for remineralization, conventional therapy must be reconsidered. For example, Bille and Thylstrup (1982) have demonstrated that more than half of the carious lesions appearing radiographically to require treatment had no macroscopic cavitation. Along the same lines, Gröndahl (1979) reported that more than one third of the lesions diagnosed as enamel caries did not extend beyond the dentinoenamel junction over a 6-year period. Along with the declining caries prevalence in adolescents, progression of proximal lesions is very

Figs 2-4a and 2-4b Bitewing radiographs are indispensable for complete diagnosis of proximal caries.

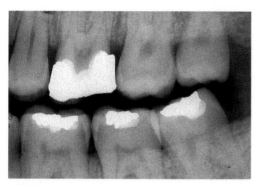

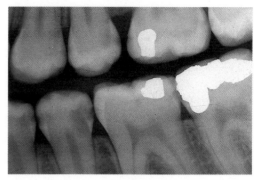

Fig 2-4a Caries has progressed into the dentin mesially and distally on the mandibular left first molar and mesially on the mandibular left second molar. The lesion on the mesial surface of the maxillary left second molar has already reached dentin. The overhanging restoration on the maxillary left second premolar may have led to minor loss of vertical height of the distal interproximal bone.

Fig 2-4b Profound caries is diagnosed distally on the mandibular left first premolar, mesially and distally on the mandibular left second premolar, and distally on the maxillary left second premolar. The lesions are localized in dentin and in the case of the mandibular second premolar, the lesion reaches the inner part of dentin. Caries is limited to the enamel on the mandibular first molar mesially and distally, the maxillary first premolar distally, the maxillary first molar mesially and distally, and the maxillary second molar mesially. This patient's average risk for caries, as expressed by a mutans streptococci concentration of greater than 10^6 colony-forming units per milliliter of saliva, indicates that the dentist should restore these enamel lesions rather than attempt remineralization.

slow. In a recent prospective study, proximal lesions that had reached the dentin increased from 1% to 14% over a 10-year period, but only 4% had spread in the outer half and less than 1% in the inner part of the dentin (Mejàre et al 1998). Thus, the choice between a preventive and a curative procedure is no longer simple. Help may be provided by estimation of the existing caries risk.

If the patient refuses radiographs, a fiberoptic transillumination (FOTI) unit may be used instead. Cold light escapes through a 0.5-mm-wide right-angled tip that is specially narrowed for the proximal spaces. Healthy dental hard tissue permits passage of light entering below the contact area, so that enamel, the dentinoenamel junction, and dentin can be identified from the occlusal surface (Figs 2-5a and 2-5b). If a carious lesion has destroyed the integrity of the crystalline structure, however, exiting light is interrupted; a carious lesion appears as a dark shadow.

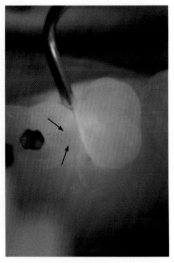

Fig 2-5a Examination for proximal caries with the Fleximed device. The distoproximal surface of the maxillary right second premolar is free of caries; proximal caries is present on the first molar mesially (arrows).

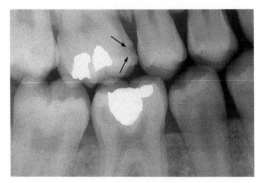

Fig 2-5b The bitewing radiograph of the same patient as in Fig 2-5a confirms the presence of proximal caries on the first molar mesially (arrows).

According to Mitropoulos (1985), in comparison with bitewing radiographs, 73% of all proximal lesions involving dentin can be identified by this procedure. Stephen et al (1986), in contrast, found only a 50% correspondence in their examination of 53,000 proximal surfaces.

Fiberoptic transillumination has several problems and disadvantages:

1. The dentist's experience is an important factor; diagnoses should be calibrated through comparison with bitewing radiographs and after therapeutic intervention.

2. It is tempting to diagnose any irregularity as caries, leading to overestimation of caries and overtreatment.

3. Restored proximal surfaces on adjacent teeth can lead to false interpretation; amalgam restorations prevent the passage of light and reflect it to the enamel of the adjacent tooth, so that light fragmentation may elicit shadows although no caries is present. This effect can be prevented by placing a white finishing strip against the amalgam restoration.

4. Excessively high light intensity leads to misinterpretation. Too little light precludes passage of the light through the dental hard tissue and may produce only a weak shadow in the presence of a carious lesion; the lesion may not be recognized.

5. Proper placement of the tip is important; the light beam must impinge on the hard tissue below the contact point in all instances.

6. As a rule, only those lesions that have reached the dentinoenamel junction are recognized; enamel lesions usually are not detected.

7. Unlike bitewing radiographs, fiberoptic transillumination does not provide other diagnostic information, such as the presence of recurring caries or secondary caries at restorations.

8. No permanent documentation of the findings is produced.

DETERMINATION OF THE EXISTING CARIES RISK

Recent epidemiologic studies have demonstrated that caries prevalence in industrialized nations is subject to increasing polarization, ie, most restorations are present in a few individuals (Marthaler 1975, Downer 1984, Hugoson et al 1988). Such polarization has been especially obvious in those nations that have already achieved significant successes in caries reduction as a result of their organized programs of prevention. According to the US National Survey of 1986/1987, approximately 30% of all 5- to 17-year-old children accounted for 87% of all decayed, missing, or filled surfaces (calculated from data in NIDR 1989). Similar relationships also have been found for Germany (Dünninger and Pieper 1991).

A study by Øgaard (1989a), comparing orthodontically treated children to untreated children, similarly found that the numbers of filled surfaces in the groups were distributed unevenly. Furthermore, these restorations often were located on surfaces that are not normally sites of caries predilection, for example, on the proximal surfaces of anterior teeth and the buccal surfaces of posterior teeth. Øgaard (1989) proposed that patients at high risk for caries be identified so that an increase in caries could be impeded during orthodontic treatment.

Subjective evaluation

Experienced practitioners, in particular, continue to claim that they can estimate precisely whether a patient is especially at risk for caries by visual inspection alone. In fact, a longitudinal study has shown that, at least over a short term (16 months), subjective evaluation of caries by an expe-

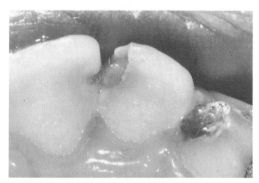

Fig 2-6 Soft caries (caries alba) indicates a high caries activity, as does the location of the lesion in the anterior tooth.

rienced dentist is a reliable indicator for caries prognosis (Heintze 1991) (Fig 2-6). Heintze proposed classification of the carious activity of the entire dentition into four categories, according to the clinical appearance of the carious lesions.

Similarly, a comprehensive 3-year study at the University of North Carolina revealed that the subjective estimation by the examiner of the anticipated increase in caries activity is among the strongest predictors of caries, together with the morphology of the pits and fissures and the initial caries prevalence (Disney et al 1992). Another common procedure for estimation of caries risk is the counting of carious lesions, which is expressed as the decayed, missing, or filled teeth (or surfaces) index. Most prevention programs are based on such estimations.

Various studies, some of which were retrospective, have indicated that the number of carious lesions is, in fact, a good predictor of a later increase in a patient's rate of caries (Honkala et al 1984, Seppä et al 1989, Wilson and Ashley 1989). Other studies have demonstrated exactly the opposite (Birkeland et al 1976, Rise et al 1979). Presumably, estimation of the number of initial carious lesions is better suited to caries prognosis. Klock and Krasse (1979) studied 300 9- to 12-year-old children and found that those children with 11 or more initial lesions at the beginning of the study had a higher rate of increase of caries activity. The high caries-predictive value of this indicator was confirmed later by Seppä and Hausen (1988b).

It is common sense, however, to predict a high probability of future increase in caries when the dentition is already seriously diseased with caries. It is far more useful to estimate the risk of caries as precisely as possible before the lesions have manifested themselves, particularly because a change in the factors causing caries can lead to cessation of carious activity in a formerly active dentition.

Diagnostic tests

The risk of caries can be determined by screening tests, with which subjects likely to become affected in the future are identified from among a large group of apparently healthy people. The diagnostic test, in contrast, is used, together with the history and the clinical symptoms, to formulate a diagnosis in the presence of manifest disease. If a screening test were incorporated in a caries prevention concept, preventive measures would be more effective because those at greatest risk could be placed into special precautionary programs.

On the individual level, diagnostic tests of caries risk also are useful, but false-positive and false-negative results must be anticipated.

In fact, various testing procedures to identify children who are allegedly at high risk for caries were developed in the past.

These tests are based predominantly on quantitative estimation of cariogenic flora and on determination of the quantity and quality of saliva.

Estimation of mutans streptococci

Despite numerous reports of a positive correlation between the presence of mutans streptococci (MS) and an increased rate of caries, the predictiveness of mutans streptococci determinations has not proven significantly better than the record of previous caries experience (review Pienihäkkinen et al 1987, Krasse 1988). A 16-month longitudinal study of 9- to 10-year-olds in Berlin indicated that the MS estimation is relatively insignificant as an explanation of caries incidence in a multifactorial model (Heintze et al 1991).

The results of numerous studies, however, show in general that the MS test identifies those patients with a low caries risk (Kingman et al 1988). If relatively few or no MS are present (negative test), it may be assumed with high probability that the patient is unlikely to develop new carious lesions. Despite this finding, the test is not predictive in the prognosis of caries for an individual patient (Seppä and Hausen 1988a, Loesche 1990). Although mutans streptococci are held to be the principal caries-inducing organisms, their quantitative estimation has only a relatively minor predictive value, which appears to be greater up to the age of 5 or 6 years (Alaluusua et al 1987) than in later years (Pienihäkkinen 1990).

False-positive results may be anticipated in youths and adults; that is, although mutans streptococci have been shown to be present in large numbers, the rate of caries is not greatly increased. What is the explanation for this, inasmuch as this group of bacteria is believed to be the principal cause of caries?

1. Oral hygiene measures and fluorida-tion measures can weaken the caries-inducing action of MS. Frequent application of low-dose fluoride sup-ports remineralization; thus, a high MS count need not necessarily lead to active carious lesions.

2. Mutans streptococci bacteria are not the sole organisms causing caries. This species includes numerous sub-groups, of which mainly two are found in humans: *Streptococcus so-brinus* and *Streptococcus mutans.* These species, however, form differ-ent amounts of acid. The MS test pro-vides no information about which type of MS organisms are present. In addition, lactobacilli also produce high amounts of acid, contributing to caries formation. Finally, the growth of other streptococci, eg, *Streptococcus sanguis,* can falsify the test result.

3. If a population group has a low caries rate on average, it is more difficult to identify those individuals with a rela-tively greater rate of caries. In con-trast, the test will be more specific in populations with a high caries preva-lence. This relationship exists for all testing procedures.

Despite its uncertain individual corre-lation, the MS test can provide useful indi-cations of a possible caries risk, particularly when it is used in very young children.

Procedures. A simple test procedure to determine mutans streptococci in the or-dinary dental practice has been developed by Jensen and Bratthall (1989). Dentocult SM (Strip mutans) is a further develop-ment of the spatula method of Köhler and Bratthall (1979). The test is based on the fact that mutans streptococci adhere not only to tooth surfaces but also to wooden or plastic spatulas and removable devices (Figs 2-7a to 2-7d).

For the test, the patient chews paraf-fin wax to stimulate the flow of saliva, rins-ing mutans streptococci from their ecological niches. A plastic spatula, rough-ened on one side, is coated with saliva by placing it under the patient's tongue sev-eral times. To remove excess saliva, the spatula is withdrawn from the mouth through the patient's lightly closed lips.

The spatula is placed in a glass tube containing fluid medium, to which a baci-tracin tablet has been added about 20 minutes beforehand. Bacitracin inhibits growth of almost all bacteria except mu-tans streptococci. The tube, with its plastic spatula, is incubated for 2 days at 37°C.

Determination of bacterial growth during this period is made with the aid of a model chart. What matters is not the size of the colonies but their density (number). Because specific microbiologic knowledge is not required, the test can be adminis-tered and evaluated by the dentist or by auxiliaries.

The threshold value for above-aver-age possibility of caries is assumed to be more than 250,000 colony-forming units (CFU) per milliliter of saliva. Values greater than 1,000,000 CFU/mL indicate a high risk of caries in all instances (Zickert et al 1982). In the Dentocult SM test, class 2 corresponds to approximately 250,000 CFU and class 3 corresponds to approxi-mately 1,000,000 CFU of MS per milli-liter saliva. However, the test result must be interpreted in relation to the number of teeth present. A result indicating class 1 in a patient with only four teeth is different from a similar result in one who has a complete dentition.

The Dentocult SM test correlates well with conventional neurobiological cultiva-tion. If it is run on different days for the

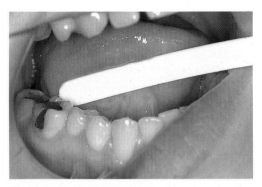

Fig 2-7a A plastic spatula is placed under the tongue and moistened with saliva.

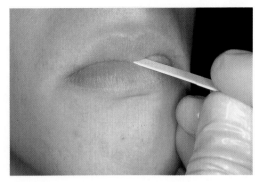

Fig 2-7b Excess saliva is removed by drawing the spatula through the patient's lightly closed lips.

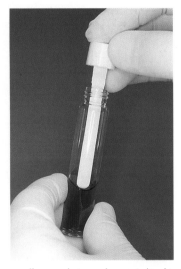

Fig 2-7c The saliva-moistened spatula is mounted in the screw closure and inserted along with a bacitracin tablet into the prepared broth.

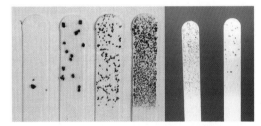

Fig 2-7d After a 2-day incubation, the density of mutans streptococci on the spatula is compared with the model chart (right to left): class $0 = 0$ to 10^3 CFU/mL; class $1 = 10^3$ to 10^5 CFU/mL; class $2 = 10^5$ to 10^6 CFU/mL; class 3 = more than 10^6 CFU/mL of saliva. The examples (on the red background) show class 2 (left) and class 1 (right) results.

same patient, differences in results may occur, but these are of a single class at most (El-Nadeef and Bratthall 1991). Because only a crude estimate of the numbers of mutans streptococci (few or many) is necessary, the above-mentioned shortcomings of the test can be ignored.

Cleaning of the teeth before the test has only a minor effect on the outcome. However, if the patient uses an oral rinse that contains chlorhexidine, that use should be discontinued 10 days before the test, because chlorhexidine interferes with adhesion of the organisms to the plastic spatula.

Occasionally, other bacteria, such as enterococci, may bleach the nutrient solution and the colonies on the plastic spatula so that it becomes difficult to recognize the colonization on the test spatula (El-Nadeef et al 1992). This problem can be avoided by adding a plaque-disclosing solution, eg, erythrosin, or by using a magnifying glass.

Streptococcal varieties other than MS can grow on the test spatula. In the case of *S sanguis,* they can be identified easily because they grow as black colonies, in contrast to the frosty blue color of MS colonies.

The test procedure also is suitable for determining MS in plaque of specific tooth surfaces (Wallmann and Krasse 1993). For this purpose, a wooden toothpick is used to scrape plaque from the tooth and transfer it to the rough surface of the plastic spatula. After 2 days of incubation, MS growth, if present, is visible on the inoculated surface. In this way, the presence of MS on high-risk surfaces and on bracket bases can be determined, and the local effect of antimicrobial measures can be assessed.

Estimation of lactobacilli

Like mutans streptococci, lactobacilli are organisms closely involved in the forma-tion of caries. Presumably they do not have a direct role in the etiology of caries but rather use existing lesions for their growth. These organisms may, however, be present before initial carious lesions have formed (Leverett et al 1993). High levels of lactobacilli indicate frequent and large consumption of carbohydrates, disaccharides in particular, and thus are a sign of increased caries risk. Estimation of the number of lactobacilli present is the oldest and best known test for caries activity (review Socransky 1968).

Procedures. Determination of lactobacilli in saliva became an office procedure in the 1970s with the introduction of a simple dip slide test (Dentocult LB) (Larmas 1975) (Figs 2-8a and 2-8b). As with the mutans streptococcus test, the patient chews paraffin wax. After 1 minute, the patient is told to swallow the saliva elicited by the chewing and to continue to chew, spitting the fresh saliva into a beaker. Collection of about 1 mL of saliva is necessary to coat both sides of the agar dip slide on which the lactobacilli are to grow. Depending on the patient's salivary flow rate, 1 to 3 minutes are required. It may be difficult to collect the required volume from small children.

The dip slide is coated with Rogosa selective *Lactobacillus agar;* this substrate selectively supports growth of acid-forming and acid-resistant lactobacilli, *Lactobacillus casei* and *Lactobacillus fermentum* in particular. Growth of most other salivary organisms is inhibited. Coating of the slide is best accomplished with a disposable syringe. Both sides of the slide must be coated completely to ensure that lactobacilli can grow on the entire dip slide, as is required for counting and evaluation against the comparison chart. Excess saliva is discarded. The dip slide is placed into the transport tube, which is closed tightly and incubated for 4 days at 37°C.

Evaluation is similar to the procedure used in the MS test. Total growth on the agar is considered. Lactobacilli form white or transparent, sharply defined colonies of varying size, depending on density. Occasionally, yeasts such as *Candida* may grow on the agar. These yeasts can be recognized through the absence of a lactic acid odor when the tube is opened and by their morphology, since *Candida* form diffuse, flat, not sharply demarcated colonies.

As in the MS test, the number, rather than the size of the colonies, is the important factor. Values greater than 100,000 CFU/mL (see Fig 2-8b) indicate an increased risk of caries (Crossner 1981). If the two sides of the dip slide show different growths, the side with the greater colony density is selected for evaluation. A study in which 10 dentists independently evaluated photographs of agar carriers with the comparison chart produced an agreement rate of nearly 80%; when two classifications were combined, eg, 1 and 2, 3 and 4, the agreement rate increased further (Heintze and Roulet 1992).

The lactobacillus test, like the MS test, serves as an indicator of low caries risk (Klock and Krasse 1979, Crossner 1981). In particular, the presence of lactobacilli reflects high consumption of carbohydrates and therefore is only an indirect test for caries. However, the test is an excellent means of checking a patient's nutritional habits (Crossner 1981, Wikner 1986). The test also provides information about the activity of existing carious lesions. High levels of lactobacillus indicate elevated carious activity and may lead to early treatment of the lesions.

Among all saliva tests, the Dentocult LB test provided the clearest indication of

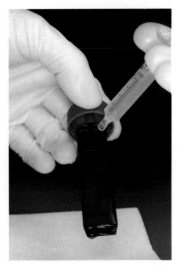

Fig 2-8a The saliva is transferred dropwise with a disposable syringe onto the dip slide.

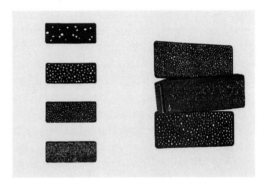

Fig 2-8b The density of lactobacillus colonies is compared to a model chart (left, top to bottom): class 1 = 103 CFU/mL; class 2 = 104 CFU/mL; class 3 = 105 CFU/mL; class 4 = 106 CFU/mL of saliva. (right) An example, placed between two model charts, shows a class 3 result.

high caries risk (Heintze et al 1991) (Table 2-1). However, in this medium-term study, initial caries prevalence (3.8 tooth surfaces) and the rate of increase in caries after 16 months (3.4 surfaces), were both relatively high. In a multifactorial statistical model, the lactobacillus test correlated and concurred strongly with two similarly definitive caries predictors: initial caries

Table 2-1 Caries predictors in a multifactorial model F-value

Type of caries	12.1
Lactobacilli test	9.8
Initial caries prevalence	6.4
Mutans streptococci test	4.6
Buffer capacity of saliva	3.0
Sucrose intake	0.2
Saliva flow rate	0.0
Stochastic variable	2.2

prevalence and the subjective evaluation of the examiner (caries type: acute vs chronic caries).

The prognosis for caries becomes more certain when the results of the MS test and the lactobacillus test are combined (Stecksén-Blicks 1985). The colonization pattern of both tests can be preserved for long periods; the lactobacillus test in a cooler for 1 year and the MS test in a dried state for as many as 10 years. The storage of specimens permits comparison with subsequent test results. If patients perceive the bacteria as their personal enemies, display of test results and comparison with earlier tests can contribute significantly to patient motivation. The patient with a high lactobacilli value may be given the opportunity to sniff the agar carrier. The patient will not soon forget the lactic acid smell and will seek to reduce the number of lactobacilli in his or her mouth through alterations in nutritional behavior (Crossner and Unell 1986).

Assessment of salivary factors

The carious process takes place in close proximity to saliva. Therefore, testing of the saliva in some manner to determine the caries risk seems logical. Determination of specific salivary enzymes and ions is difficult. In contrast, measurement of the volume of saliva per time unit (salivary flow rate) and salivary buffer capacity is simple.

Flow rate. In theory, it seems clear that a high salivary flow rate would inhibit the growth of MS and its adhesion to the tooth surface. In fact, such an effect has been shown. Yet it has not been possible to demonstrate clearly that a definite relationship exists between the volume of saliva and the development of caries (Klock and Krasse 1979, Heintze 1991). Only in patients with xerostomia, whose salivary flow is significantly reduced as a consequence of partial destruction of the salivary glands, has it been possible to establish an increased caries rate (Dreizen and Brown 1976).

Because the salivary flow rate varies greatly among patients, it can only round out the picture of the caries risk. That the flow rate can be established easily and without any special devices is a great advantage. Thus, the saliva collected for the lactobacillus test can be used to measure the salivary flow rate as well.

Stimulated salivary flow of less than 0.7 mL/min is considered low for adults; values higher than 1.0 mL/min are considered normal. As a rule, women have slightly smaller salivary glands than men, so that their salivary flow rate is slightly lower. Similarly, children have a lower salivary flow rate than adolescents and adults because their salivary glands are not fully formed yet.

The results of these measurements may be affected by the patient's drug intake. Certain kinds of drugs inhibit the flow rate: anticholinergic agents (for intestinal tract disturbances); antihistamines (for allergies); sedatives; and neuroleptic agents (for neurologic illness, eg, schizophrenia). Other agents, such as appetite suppressants, antihypertensive medications, those that stimulate production of urine, and cytotoxic drugs, also may inhibit salivary flow. Some of these drugs are taken as antistress medications, leading to a vicious circle, because stress itself reduces salivary flow as a consequence of adrenaline secretion and other factors.

Buffer capacity. The buffer capacity indicates the extent to which the salivary buffer systems can neutralize acids. The lower the pH at the end of a measurement, the greater and more enduring is the effect of the acids produced by the bacteria.

The buffer capacity of saliva can be measured easily with the Dentobuff strip test. A disposable syringe is used to place a single drop of paraffin-stimulated saliva on a test strip. After about 5 minutes, the color change on the pH indicator strip is compared with the color chart provided (Fig 2-9).

The determination of buffer capacity, like that of the salivary flow rate, has only a subordinate role in the reliable identification of patients at high risk for caries.

The buffer capacity test has greater value in patients with exposed root surfaces, because exposed dentin is more sensitive to acid than enamel.

Enzymes and ions. An investigation by Leverett and coworkers indicated that the degree of saturation of fluoroapatite and phosphate ion of saliva, together with determination of mutans streptococci and lactobacilli, appears to be strongly caries predictive; caries development over the succeeding 12 months was predicted correctly in more than 80% of the 6-year-olds

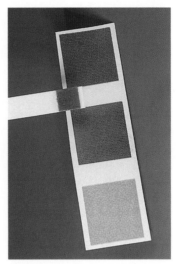

Fig 2-9 The buffer capacity of a saliva sample is evaluated with the aid of a test strip.

examined (Leverett et al 1993). In accordance with the etiology of caries, it is reasonable to evaluate cariogenic (bacterial) and protective (fluoroapatite) factors to estimate the actual risk of caries with some certainty. If the protective mechanisms are sufficiently strong, caries progression can be stopped even when mutans streptococci and lactobacilli are present in large numbers.

Measurement of plaque

Among all indices related in any way to plaque, the plaque formation rate index (PFRI) has been found to be particularly useful in predicting increases in the rate of caries (Axelsson 1991). The PFRI measures the speed with which new plaque grows. Plaque formed in the 24-hour period following a professional tooth cleaning is evaluated with a five-level scale. The patient must refrain from brushing the teeth during the test period. The percentage of affected tooth surfaces is calculated according to the formula:

$$\frac{\text{Total number of surfaces with plaque} \times 100}{\text{Number of teeth} \times 6 \text{ (surfaces per tooth)}}$$

The result is compared with a five-point scale (Table 2-2).

The PFRI is used to evaluate the total effect of the various influences (salivary flow rate, salivary glycoproteins, quality and quantity of the microflora, fermentable carbohydrates, etc) affecting plaque formation. Longitudinal studies have shown the PFRI to have a strong predictive value, which can be increased by combination with the mutans streptococci estimation (Axelsson 1991). A PFRI of III or greater in the presence of simultaneously high MS levels is associated with high caries prevalence (Axelsson 1990). However, determination of this index is relatively time consuming, because the patient must be examined on 2 consecutive days.

Caries risk formula

A responsible dentist cannot rely exclusively on any single test, but must take as many factors as possible into consideration when estimating the risk of progression of caries. It is sensible to make estimates of the risk of caries at specific intervals. In this way, the dentist can complete his or her understanding of a patient's caries condition through a series of analyses that depict the condition at particular moments over a period of time. Only in that way does the dentist know the present (and perhaps altered) caries risk. The effectiveness of individual intensive preventive measures also should be checked on the basis of the tests described previously.

In principle, all considerations aimed at evaluation of the caries risk should take the prevalence of caries in the population involved into account. As already noted, it is far more difficult, according to Klock et al (1989), to identify patients at high risk in a population with a low caries rate.

On the level of the individual patient, success or failure of the dentist's oral hygiene efforts depends on the reliable appraisal of the risk of caries. Suhonen and Tenovuo (1989) attempted to reduce the individual's risk of caries to the formula:

$$\text{Caries risk} = S \text{ mutans} \times \frac{\text{Sucrose intake}}{\text{Defense mechanisms}}$$

According to this formula, the caries risk is highest when the intake of sucrose is high, S mutans has a favorable environmental niche in the oral cavity, and various defense factors either are absent or ineffective. If sucrose uptake is low and defense mechanisms are strong, however, the caries risk may be low despite the presence of large numbers of S mutans.

Table 2-2 The five levels of PFRI measuring the proportion of plaque accumulation

PFRI level	Plaque formation on tooth surfaces (%)	Characteristic
I	1–10	very low
II	11–20	low
III	21–30	middle
IV	31–40	high
V	>40	very high

DIAGNOSIS OF PERIODONTITIS

The inflammatory loss of periodontal ligament is a common disease with high prevalence worldwide (Miyazaki et al 1991a and 1991b). Prevalence increases with age, but there are early-onset types of periodontitis that already affect adolescents and young adults (Ranney 1993). The latest nationwide survey showed for the US that over 90% of individuals 13 years and older had experienced loss of attachment, but only 15% exhibited severe destruction (loss of attachment greater than 5 mm) (Brown et al 1996). Only 6.4% of the 25- to 34-year-old Americans had attachment loss of 5 mm or greater; in the 35–44 age group the percentage is 12.3. Localized juvenile periodontitis (LJP), characterized by significant rapid bone loss in the region of the incisors and first molars, has a prevalence of 0.53% in US adolescents—according to a survey carried out in the 1980s (Löe and Brown 1991). Black males are about three times as likely to have LJP as black females, whereas in the white population females are affected three times more often than males. Generalized juvenile periodontitis occurs only in 0.13% of all adolescents.

Periodontal disease is the clinical result of a complex interaction between the host and plaque bacteria (Genco 1996). Although found for *Actinobacillus actinomycetemcomitans* in prepubertal and juvenile periodontitis, and to some degree for the rapidly progressive periodontitis, it has been difficult to obtain evidence for a specific etiological role of bacteria associated with periodontal disease in adults. What is seen is the net result of host-parasite interactions which in an unpredictable moment accumulates and exceeds the threshold of tissue integrity. The course of periodontal breakdown (bursts, continuous development, velocity) is determined by the reaction of the host. The expression of periodontal disease has a strong genetic component, which presumably defines the host's response thereby affecting susceptibility (Offenbacher et al 1993a). The risk associated with periodontal disease progression is primarily patient-based and secondarily site-based. Some microorganisms (risk markers) occur more frequently than others and may significantly determine the outcome of this host-parasite interaction (Dahlén 1993).

Assessment of Periodontitis Risk

People of all ages develop periodontal diseases to a varying extent. Some regions of the dentition (for example, the maxillary molars) are more frequently and more severely affected. The development and progression of periodontitis arise from the interplay of periodontopathic bacteria and the host's immune defense system. Science has long sought a diagnostic procedure to predict the risk of periodontitis through determination of the attack and defense mechanisms, for clinical parameters are not sufficient to accurately identify patients with potential disease activity. Therefore overtreatment is a likely possibility. Periodontal diseases are under growing scrutiny from the medical profession because of their possible link to systemic diseases such as cardiovascular diseases (eg, endocarditis; Herzberg and Meyer 1996; Kweider et al 1993). Also, they have a potentially aggravating effect on diabetes symptoms (Genco 1996, Taylor et al 1996, Thorstensson et al 1996). Further, they may play a role as an etiological cofactor for lower birth-weight

(Papapanou 1996; Slavkin 1997). Therefore, the identification of people at risk to develop periodontitis is of superior importance. Finally, there is evidence that periodontitis-associated bacteria or their tissue-derived inflammatory mediators are transmitted during pregnancy from mother to child (Slavkin 1997). To prevent such transmission by adequate therapy (mechanical debridement, antibiotics), accurate diagnostic tests are needed.

Risk markers that might provide information on the prognosis of periodontitis include the search for substances that are associated with bacteria (eg, DNA-analysis, assessment of antigen profile, enzymatic activity), specific enzymes involved in tissue breakdown (eg, aspartate aminotransferase, collagenoses) as well as inflammatory mediators (interleukin; review Armitage 1992).

Numerous chairside tests are available that measure different parameters associated with periodontitis development. However, it still is not clear to what extent the results of these tests are clinically significant. According to several recently published reviews, none of the already available tests is capable of identifying with at least 80% accuracy those individuals that are at risk for periodontitis (Greenstein 1994, Jeffcoat et al 1997, Lamster 1997, Lamster et al 1993, Lang and Brägger 1991).

Microbial testing has proven to have some benefit in medically compromised patients, in early-onset periodontitis patients, and in refractory periodontitis patients (Jeffcoat et al 1997). However, in these individuals antimicrobial therapy may be indicated, regardless of the outcome of periodontal tests.

As far as biochemical profiles in the gingival crevicular fluid are concerned, some value has been attributed to the measurement of aspartate aminotransferase (Persson and Page 1992), β-glucoronidase (Lamster et al 1993), and prostaglandin E2 (Offenbacher et al 1993b). A combined test that takes into account both the bacterial challenge and the host response may possess satisfactory predictive power for screening subjects at risk as well as for patients in the posttreatment phase.

Therefore, clinical evaluation is still the most pragmatic, though not the most accurate, way to carry out periodontal diagnosis and risk assessment:

1. Does gingival bleeding appear in response to careful probing?
2. Do periodontal pockets exist? How deep are they?
3. Are alterations of bone apparent on radiographs (periapical, bitewing, panoramic)?

Clinical measurements

What clinical parameters are available for the diagnosis of progressive periodontitis? Haffajee et al (1991) concluded, from their longitudinal study, that only the visible plaque and bleeding in response to probing are related to progressive periodontitis; the patient's age is an additional risk factor. Bleeding as such, however, is not a perfect diagnostic instrument. A study by Lang et al (1990) indicated progressive disease in only 6% of those with bleeding. Not bleeding, however, is a reliable indicator for periodontal health since 98% of non-bleeding sites do not develop periodontal breakdown.

These observations permit the conclusion that a nonbleeding periodontium is and will remain healthy, even in the presence of a periodontal pocket. In contrast, bleeding alone does not indicate loss of attachment, even if this stability is not the same as periodontal health. Bleeding always is an indication of inflammation. Although such inflammation can remain in equilibrium, if the balance between attack and resistance factors is tipped in favor of disease, loss of attachment is unavoidable.

Gingival bleeding index

Use of an index is necessary to check the course of periodontitis. The gingival bleeding index is simple, yet efficient (Ainamo and Bay 1975). The sulcus is probed carefully on the facial and lingual surfaces with a periodontal probe (Fig 2-10). It is useful to develop a specific system for this purpose, eg, to proceed by quadrants. Probing begins on the facial surface, proceeding from the distal to the mesial surface, then on the lingual surface from the distal to the mesial. Thus each tooth has four points of measurement: facial, lingual, mesioproximal, and distoproximal.

The presence or absence of bleeding is noted on a prepared form. Every bleeding site is inflamed and deserves attention, regardless of the degree of bleeding. The

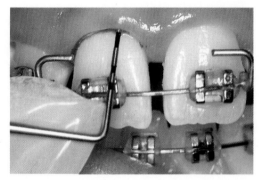

Fig 2-10 The sulcus is examined with a periodontal probe to determine the gingival bleeding index.

percentage of bleeding sites is calculated as a percentage of all sites measured. Figure 2-11 presents an example together with the relevant calculations.

Probing is difficult in patients with fixed appliances, because bands and other attachments limit access to the gingival margin (Figs 2-12; 2-13a and 2-13b). Still, it is necessary to probe the gingival margin along its entire length; a certain amount of patience and experience is required.

$$\frac{\text{Number of bleeding sites}}{\text{Total number of sites}} \times 100 = \% \text{ gingivitis}$$

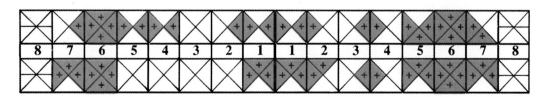

$$\frac{53}{112} \times 100 = 47\% \text{ gingivitis}$$

Fig 2-11 Example of the Ainamo's Gingival Bleeding Index. The sulcus of each tooth is probed. Four sites are measured: facial, lingual, mesioproximal, and distoproximal. The presence or absence of bleeding at each site is noted.

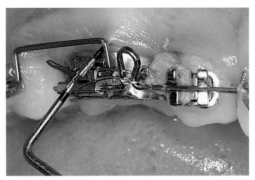

Fig 2-12 A segmented arch between the maxillary right first and second molars impedes periodontal probing. The same is true for the rotation module distal to the second premolar.

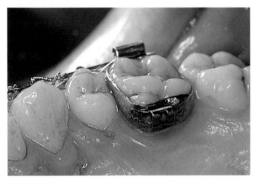

Fig 2-13a The transpalatial arch tube at the maxillary right first molar impedes good oral hygiene, leading to inflammation of the periodontium.

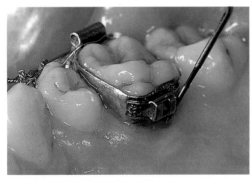

Fig 2-13b The lingual attachment makes periodontal probing difficult.

Loss of attachment

The principal symptom of periodontitis is the loss of tooth-supporting structures with the formation of gingival and infrabony pockets. The periodontal examination therefore requires documentation of the loss of attachment. For this purpose, the pocket is probed gently with a measuring probe to the floor of the pocket. The sulcus is maximally 0.5 mm deep in a histologically sound gingiva. A probe can measure depths up to 2.5 mm, because it intrudes into the junctional epithelium. Where periodontitis exists, the probe reaches as deeply as the first fibers that extend into the root cementum. As a consequence, clinical measurements exceed anatomic-histologic findings by 0.5 to 2.0 mm.

Pressure cannot be completely eliminated during any such measurement, leading to a systematic error. So that, at the least, reproducible measurements can be obtained, probes that, when used properly, fix pressure at 0.2 to 0.4 N have been developed (eg, Florida Probe). The reference point (gingival margin [GM] or cementoenamel junction [CEJ]) must be set manually at the beginning of the measurement. The results are recorded and may be stored in a computer.

Tipping of the probe affects the precision of the measurements, but the problem can be overcome by tip sensors, available on some systems. One probe (Jeffcoat et al 1986) not only includes such a sensor but also automatically determines the position of the CEJ, providing an important parameter for calculation of attachment loss.

The probing depth alone provides information only about existing reduction of the height of the periodontal fibers in relation to the height of the gingival margin. It is not a measure of the possible loss of attachment. For example, probing depth does not reflect gingival recession or gingival hyperplasia. In the presence of gingival recession, measurement of probing depth would indicate too little loss of attachment; in the presence of gingival hyperplasia, the loss would be exaggerated. If the primary interest is the loss of periodontal attachment, the distance between the height of the GM and the CEJ must be measured.

To determine this measurement, the probing depth must be added in the case of gingival recession and subtracted in the case of a pseudopocket. Two examples illustrate this calculation:

1. Probing depth = 4 mm
GM – CEJ = 2 mm (because of gingival recession)
Attachment loss = 4 mm + 2 mm = 6 mm

2. Probing depth = 5 mm
GM – CEJ = 2 mm (because of the existence of a pseudopocket)
Attachment loss = 5 mm – 2 mm = 3 mm

The remaining attachment (attachment level) depends, in the final analysis, on the length and thickness of the roots and can be evaluated only in conjunction with a radiograph. The radiograph provides information about the height of the alveolar bone, vertical pockets, and apical periodontal disease.

But the measurement of attachment loss does not correlate with the inflammatory activity of a pocket and is therefore not an adequate tool for risk assessment (Lang and Corbet 1995).

Epidemiologic data

In addition to clinical and radiographic parameters, epidemiologic data provide information about groups at higher risk for periodontitis (Fox 1992):

1. Smokers
2. Diabetics
3. Patients with osteoporosis
4. Persons who neglect oral hygiene
5. Patients with previous periodontal disease
6. Elderly persons

Prognosis

The prognosis of an existing periodontitis is complicated due to the fact that the course of this disease is more likely to be episodic. However, with more accurate probes that operate with a precision of 0.2 mm, it has been possible to demonstrate experimentally that, contrary to classic academic belief, periodontal breakdown is usually continuous (67%), rather than episodic with periods of remission (12%) (Jeffcoat and Reddy 1991). Albandar (1990) reported that more than 90% of the sites of measurement in 142 patients with periodontitis showed no increase in bone loss over a 6-year period. According to Listgarten (1986), most deep periodontal pockets never collapse completely.

At present, there is no simple and simultaneously dependable parameter or method with which it is possible to predict the progress of an existing periodontitis. The tendency to hemorrhage remains the most certain sign of periodontal destruction. Because prevention is better than healing, the clinician should take the existence of gingival bleeding very seriously and instruct the patient in an effective system of oral hygiene. Periodic removal of plaque and calculus in the critical zones, particularly in the posterior teeth, diminishes the disease in most periodontal conditions. A program of regular professional oral hygiene brings under control at-risk patients during their phases of neglect.

Professional Measures for Reducing Oral Bacteria

3

Orthodontic therapy, particularly with fixed appliances, involves the risk that functional and esthetic improvements are achieved at the cost of increases in carious activity and gingival inflammation. Orthodontic patients are likely to experience a multiplication of cariogenic and periodontopathic microorganisms, primarily because of greater accumulation of bacteria-harboring plaque. It is the responsibility of the orthodontist to involve patients in a systematic program for the prevention of caries and periodontal disease, focusing on the removal of plaque and elimination of pathologic organisms.

PROFESSIONAL TOOTH CLEANING

Professional removal of all deposits on the teeth by a dentist, dental hygienist, or specially trained assistant is considered the cornerstone of an individualized program of oral hygiene. Such tooth cleaning should be performed meticulously either manually with curettes (Fig 3-1a) or mechanically with rubber cups or brushes (Fig 3-1b) and prophylaxis paste (Figs 3-1c and 3-1d). Mineralized plaque, ie, calculus, must be removed first with manual or ultrasonic scalers (Figs 3-2a and 3-2b). Neither me-

chanical nor manual tooth cleaning reaches the proximal surfaces or the base of fissures sufficiently. Therefore, dental floss must be used interproximally, and the fissures must be sealed, if indicated.

Commonly used and critically appraised methods of professional tooth cleaning are described in the following sections. Their goal is the complete mechanical removal of microbial plaque. However, the benefits of these methods must be judged in terms of their effects on the dental hard tissues.

Effects of abrasion

Prophylaxis and polishing pastes, like toothpastes, achieve their cleaning function principally through abrasive grinding agents, eg, pumice. Medium- and coarse-grained pastes based on pumice or zirconium sulfate are preferred by dentists. With these materials, both plaque and discolorations are removed, the dentist or hygienist spending 5 seconds, on average, with each tooth.

Such pastes cause a certain amount of damage to the tooth surfaces as a consequence of their grinding action. Each abrasive, acting in concert with the hardness of the brush, the pressure and speed during its application and the heat developed thereby, the duration of the cleaning pe-

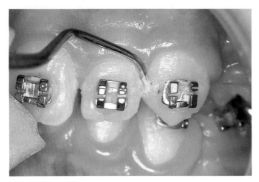

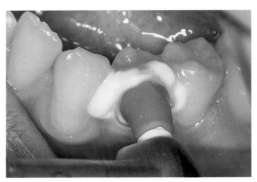

Fig 3-1a Professional removal of deposits from teeth is initiated with a curette.

Fig 3-1b Teeth should be polished only with a rubber cup and a paste containing fluoride.

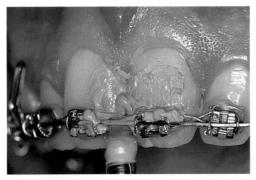

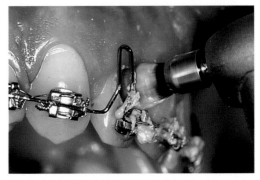

Figs 3-1c and 3-1d Polishing during a professional prophylaxis should be accomplished with a rubber cup (see Fig 3-1b) or a small brush so that the tooth surfaces under the wires can be cleaned.

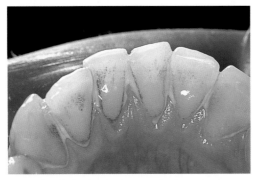

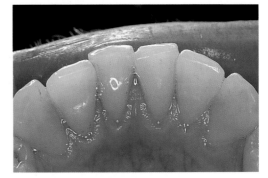

Fig 3-2a Calculus is present in the anterior region of the mandible.

Fig 3-2b Plaque has been removed with an ultrasonic unit and scalers.

riod, and the liquefaction component provided by saliva removes a certain amount of hard tissue and roughens the outer enamel. How should these two properties, cleaning and abrasion, be evaluated?

Enamel roughness

Considerable differences in the roughness of natural tooth surfaces and restorations following cleaning and polishing with various prophylaxis and polishing pastes have been reported (Roulet and Roulet-Mehrens 1982). With a single exception (Superpolish), all polishing pastes led to increased roughness. Soon after mechanical cleaning, both polished and unpolished tooth surfaces are recolonized with plaque bacteria. Therefore, according to Frandsen (1986), there is no scientifically sound evidence for a relationship between tooth surface roughness and plaque adhesion. Only visibly rough surfaces of teeth and restorations promote plaque retention decisively (Sheiham 1977). In contrast, in vivo studies have demonstrated that rough tooth surfaces promote formation of plaque (Quirynen et al 1990).

Enamel loss

In addition to the surface roughness left by any abrasive agent, the loss of dental enamel caused by the abrasivity of a polishing paste is an important factor. These two properties are related to a certain extent. The ideal prophylaxis paste, like the ideal dentifrice, should have maximum cleaning and polishing action but minimal abrasivity. If the abrasivity of a paste is low, enamel discolorations are hard to remove completely. Consequently, more time is required for cleaning.

If the root surface is exposed as a result of gingival recession, much root cementum or dentin may be removed accidentally. In general, loss of dental hard tissue is relatively small for many prophylaxis pastes. It has been found that 0.6 to 4.0 μm enamel are lost through 30 seconds of polishing, depending on the paste used, pumice being the strongest abrasive (Barbakow et al 1986). Dentin is less resistant to abrasion than enamel; the latter is 19 times more resistant to abrasion (Stookey and Schemehorn 1978).

Abrasivity of materials and instruments

Prophylaxis pastes

How is a dentist or an orthodontist to know which prophylaxis paste has what abrasivity? Some help in this direction is provided by the manufacturer through the list of cleaning agents used. The highest abrasivity is provided by pumice and zirconium sulfate, and the lowest by calcium pyrophosphate and dicalcium phosphate dihydrate (Newbrun 1989). But even pastes with the same components have different degrees of abrasiveness, even from lot to lot. These differences probably can be ascribed to variations in the concentration of the abrasive, the method of fabrication, and the various binders used (Barbakow et al 1986). The pH of a cleaning or polishing paste has an effect on abrasion, too: the lower the pH, the higher the abrasivity.

The measuring procedures accepted by the American Dental Association for determining abrasivity are radioactive dentin abrasion (RDA) and radioactive enamel abrasion (REA) (see review by Barbakow et al 1987a). The principle behind these procedures is the quantitative determination of radioactively marked dentin or enamel removed from extracted teeth by a tooth-cleaning machine and the prophylaxis paste suspension being tested.

When the cleaning procedure is completed, the radioactivity of the suspension is measured and compared with a standard suspension of calcium pyrophosphate. Many factors, particularly the dilutive and buffering effect of saliva, are ignored. Nevertheless, such numerical values simplify the choice of an appropriate prophylaxis paste for the practitioner; for that reason, RDA and REA values should be disclosed by the manufacturers. For children and adolescents, prophylaxis pastes with RDA values between 40.0 and 120.0 and REA values between 5.0 and 10.0 should be chosen.

In the case of dentifrices, the abrasiveness has a much higher importance because of daily use. Therefore, dentifrices with RDA values below 50 should be preferred (Barbakow et al 1987a).

Prophypaste System. The Prophypaste System is a prophylaxis paste system specially developed for stain removal. It is available in four grades: CCS 40 is for fine polishing, CCS 120 is for removal of plaque and discolorations, CCS 170 is for rough tooth surfaces and heavy plaque, and CCS 250 is for very rough surfaces and very heavy plaque. Each of these pastes contains sodium fluoride in addition to pumice and amorphous silicate. In use, the RDA values implied by their grade designations are not reached. According to Lutz et al (1993b), the RDA of CCS 250 was only 46.6 after a 30-second polish with a rubber cup; the REA was 12.7. Accordingly, CCS 40 is exclusively a polishing paste with no cleansing action. (The RDA after 30 seconds is 3.0; the REA is 1.8.)

Depending on the need (slight or severe staining or thick or thin plaque layer), the prophylaxis paste with the RDA (40.0 to 250.0) best suited to the condition is used first. That paste is followed by pastes of lower activity, until finally the polishing paste is used. However, this procedure appears very complicated and time consuming.

Cleanic. A universal cleaning and prophylaxis paste (Cleanic), in which the abrasive material changes in seconds from coarse grained to fine grained under the force arising from rubber cup or brush application, has been marketed. The fragile crystals of the natural abrasive perlite (concentration approximately 50%) splinter and become rounded when force is applied; furthermore, the abrasive particles become aligned parallel to the surface (Lutz et al 1993a). The RDA value of Cleanic is 25.1 with a rubber cup and 42.7 when a brush is used for 30 seconds of polishing at 2.45 N pressure at a rotational speed of 1800 rpm in a handpiece. The REA values under the same conditions are 3.4 and 6.8, respectively (Lutz et al 1993b).

These very low abrasivity values are combined in Cleanic with a level of cleaning power otherwise achieved only with prophylaxis pastes containing pumice. In addition, Cleanic smooths and polishes the surfaces of enamel and dentin satisfactorily (Lutz et al 1993b). The roughening effect of Cleanic is significantly lower than that of a dentifrice with only an average cleaning effect.

Only three teeth at a time should be treated with a single portion of Cleanic from coarse cleaning to final polish; fresh material should be used for the next group of three teeth (Fig 3-3), thus making the procedure time-consuming, too.

A prerequisite for the twofold effect (cleaning and polishing) of Cleanic is retention of the paste on the tooth surface for as long as is required for the abrasive to be ground. Because the buccal surface of a tooth bearing a bracket is divided into several individual regions, each tooth should be treated with a separate portion of Cleanic.

The previous considerations relating to abrasivity and cleaning power of various prophylaxis pastes should not be given undue importance. None of these pastes is used daily or weekly, after all, and even careful plaque removal with curettes removes a minimal amount of dental hard tissue (McCann et al 1990). Nonetheless, the dentist and the orthodontist must know these materials, especially for patients in a recall system, because the more frequent a professional tooth cleaning, the greater the possibility of gingival recession and exposure of root surfaces, even in adolescents.

Fluoridated pastes. That every polishing of the tooth carries away superficial fluoride-rich enamel layers remains a problem. For that reason, it is desirable that the polishing paste make fluoride ions available for the tooth surface. In the absence of reliable data about the bioavailability of fluoride, the caries-protective effect of such pastes is not assured (Schröder 1992). In fact, professional tooth cleaning with use of a polishing paste has a preventive effect only when provided monthly—whether the paste contains fluoride or not. As the sole source of fluoride, fluoridated prophylaxis pastes have a very limited cariostatic effect (Alexander 1980), particularly if they are used only two to four times annually during routine prophylaxis. More frequent use of prophylaxis paste is logically of greater usefulness (Stookey 1990), but that is true for all sorts of fluoride applications. Ripa (1985) has provided a comprehensive review of this topic.

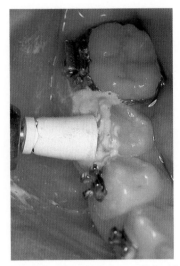

Fig 3-3 Cleanic has a self-limiting abrasive action because its abrasive changes from coarse to fine grained through pressure from a rubber cup or brush. For that reason, ideally, fresh material should be used for every three teeth.

Cleaning instruments

Rotating instruments. The contribution to enamel loss made by the cleaning device itself varies. Rotating brushes with hard bristles remove comparably more substance than do those with soft bristles, but no uniquely accepted definition of bristle hardness exists. As a whole, the differences between enamel abrasion and dentin abrasion are minor (Lutz et al 1993a). The loss of hard tissue in a single cleaning and polishing process is particularly significant because a portion of the outer enamel layer, which is rich in fluoride, is removed. In addition, some of the existing fluoroapatite is converted to calcium apatite as a result of the heat developed in the cleaning process (Alexander 1980). This conversion occurs even with rubber cups, which therefore should be used very carefully and only in combination with a minimally abrasive paste.

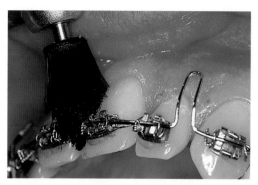

Fig 3-4 The bristles of the Rota-Dent toothbrush can be mounted in a dental contra-angle with a mandrel and clean well in the proximal spaces and around the brackets.

In principle, the use of rubber cups or rotating brushes appears superfluous after careful plaque removal by hand instruments. Plaque removal with hand instruments, however, assumes the removal of orthodontic arch wires, because the tooth surfaces otherwise are practically inaccessible. The removal of arch wires, however, is only possible in an orthodontic practice. Thus, an exclusively hand-instrumented tooth cleaning is impractical if carried out by a general dentist. For that reason, Lutz et al (1993a) proposed cleaning only with polishing brushes, without paste for children and youths, particularly because they found a relatively high cleaning power and minimal enamel abrasion with this technique.

Because an exclusively manual plaque removal is very difficult in patients with fixed appliances, and because of the above-mentioned disadvantages of brushes, the tooth surfaces must be treated with a rubber cup and a low-abrasive paste as well. Gentle but effective plaque removal, especially around the brackets, is possible with the Rota-Brush (see chapter 4). The brushes of this device can also be used in the dental handpiece (Fig 3-4).

Air polishing units. Another effective possibility for complete plaque removal from all teeth in a brief time is provided by air polishing units (eg, Prophy-Jet). When used properly, such devices are as gentle to the gingiva as is cleaning with a rubber cup and prophylaxis paste (Weaks et al 1984, Mishkin et al 1986, DeSpain and Nobis 1987, Munley et al 1987; review Jost-Brinkmann 1998) (Figs 3-5a and 3-5b). Although some authors have found no disadvantageous consequences to resin composites and amalgam (Gorfil et al 1989) or zinc phosphate cement (Barnes et al 1990), Eliades et al (1991) reported surface alterations on various restorative materials.

Although very little enamel is removed when a proper device is used (Koultan et al 1990), dentin abrasion is very high (Jost-Brinkmann 1997). Restraint is required, therefore, when pulsating devices are used on patients with exposed dentinal surfaces (Dederich et al 1989), although patients perceive these devices as more pleasant than the use of hand instruments (Clinical Research Associates 1981). Furthermore, the enamel surface is smoother after air polishing treatment than after a polish with pumice (Hannemann and Diedrich 1986, Hosoya and Johnston 1989). Air polishing provides the additional advantage of dependably eliminating plaque from uneven spots and scratches in the enamel not accessible to rotating instruments and prophylaxis paste.

Hypertension and renal disease are said to be contraindications to use of the procedure, because of the high sodium content of the sodium bicarbonate powder, even though no clinically relevant changes of arterial blood values were found in dogs after air polishing for 5 minutes (Snyder et al 1990).

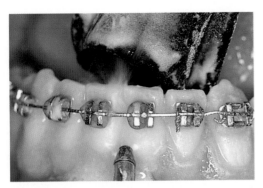

Fig 3-5a The mandibular incisors are cleaned with an air polishing unit.

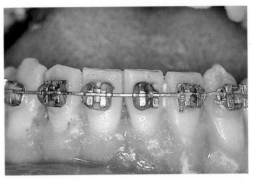

Fig 3-5b Cleaning with air polishing caused minor gingival bleeding, as is found after use of rotating instruments.

Patient reports of submucous emphysema, bone loss around implants (Bergendal et al 1990), and pneumoparotitis (Brown et al 1992) following inappropriate use of air polishing devices do not provide contraindications for their use, because the same argument could be used against all grinding instruments. It is important, however, to be aware that significant differences exist among air polishing units (Jost-Brinkmann 1998)

Effectiveness of professional prophylaxis

When professional prophylaxis is considered from the point of view of cost-benefit analysis, it is expensive. Furthermore, professional cleaning does not reduce the level of *Streptococcus mutans* in the saliva or plaque significantly (Caufield and Gibbons 1979, Emilson et al 1982). A preventive effect in terms of caries and periodontal disease can be anticipated only if these oral hygiene measures are provided in the office and home care is checked at brief intervals by professionals (Axelsson and Lindhe 1974, Poulsen et al 1976, Axelsson and Lindhe 1977, Axelsson and Lindhe 1981a, Axelsson et al 1991). The effectiveness of professional prophylaxis has been demonstrated in patients with fixed orthodontic appliances, too. A study by Alstad and Zachrisson (1979) showed that gingival inflammation is reduced in patients who had poor oral hygiene at the outset, if they are given professional cleanings at 2-week intervals. If the patients clean their teeth themselves while being watched, the reduction in gingival inflammation is less extensive (Horowitz et al 1977, Vestergaard et al 1978) or no longer observed at all (Silverstein et al 1977, Ashley and Sainsbury 1981).

Supragingival plaque removal has only a limited effect in patients with established periodontal disease (Baderstein et al 1984a, 1984b). Above all else, long-term success depends on the removal of subgingival plaque. For that reason, the effects of deep scaling and root planing on all forms of periodontitis are scientifically undisputed. Even a single instrumented removal of subgingival plaque can reduce a probing depth from 6 to 4 mm within 3 months (Baderstein et al 1984b).

If patients carry out excellent oral hygiene, no recolonization of microorganisms need be anticipated.

Because the activity of a single periodontal lesion often is not diagnosed or a dentition is simply treated in a generalized way, regardless of variously distributed disease states, the practitioner must be careful to avoid overtreatment, especially with surgical interventions. Overtreatment frequently leads to excessive loss of root dentin. A study by Baderstein et al (1984b) demonstrated clearly that nonsurgical treatment is successful in minor to advanced periodontitis. Periodontal surgery is indicated only when probing depth exceeds 6 mm and in case of recurrences (Claffey 1991). Surgical elimination of pockets is no longer the most important goal of periodontal therapy, because probing depth alone does not permit conclusions about the activity of a gingival pocket.

In terms of root planing technique, the traditional belief that all hard and soft deposits and endotoxin-infected root cementum must be removed is no longer sustainable, according to Nyman et al (1988). These authors did not find any difference in terms of periodontal health between traditional scaling and the sole use of a rubber cup and prophylaxis paste. Intentionally excessive removal of root cementum thus is superfluous or even counterproductive, because bacteria may penetrate the dentinal canals. If scaled root surfaces come to lie supragingivally, excessively sensitive cementoenamel junction may result.

RESTORATIVE METHODS

Continued monitoring of the teeth and the gingiva goes along with preventive measures, so that restorative-curative measures can be initiated promptly if necessary.

Restoration of carious lesions

All carious lesions, including those in primary teeth, must either be treated with therapeutic fluoridation, definitive restorations or other adequate measures, eg, removal of caries by grinding, therapeutic sealing, placement of prefabricated crowns, or extraction (Figs 3-6a and 3-6b). Overhanging restorations must be eliminated, and unfavorable interdental space arrangement that leads to food impaction must be avoided.

If a complete dentition has remained caries-free for 4 to 6 years, it may be classified as caries resistant. Otherwise, the weak points of the various teeth have become carious, have been restored, or remain untreated. Proximal caries is the exception to this rule. Late caries can occur here as a result of altered interdental spaces.

Clinical experience permits classification of the entire patient population into the so-called pit and fissure proximal caries types. Independently of their pathological plaque reservoir with specific cariogenic bacteria and a fermentable substrate, the pit and fissure caries group is characterized by having unfavorable anatomic fissures and pits, while the proximal caries group has pits and fissures that can be cleaned readily. The latter group, however, has unfavorably close contact of the posterior teeth as a consequence of mesial tooth migration. In the event of plaque retention, this can be a cause of extensive proximal caries.

Proximal caries provides great difficulties in diagnosis for all dentists. It is only too easy to classify a dentition as entirely

Fig 3-6a and 3-6b The mixed dentition has been restored with sealings, restorations, and stainless steel crowns. The risk of caries is now low. Orthodontic therapy can be initiated.

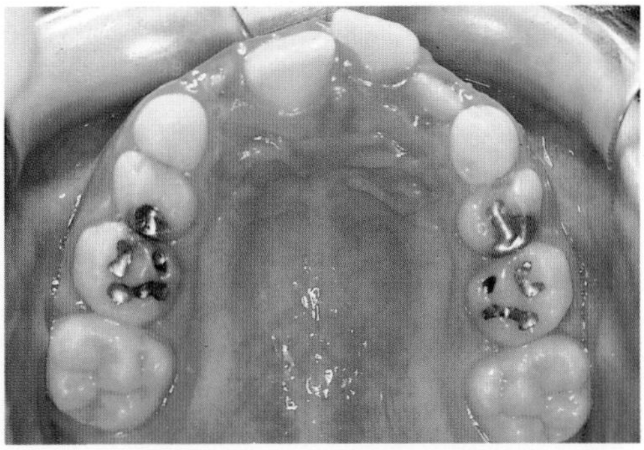

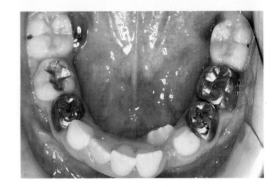

Fig 3-6a Maxilla with anterior crowding.

Fig 3-6b Mandible with ectopic eruption of the left lateral incisor.

healthy when massive loss of substance already has occurred interproximally. Often, damage is already irreversible when the occlusal margins finally fracture. For that reason, bitewing radiographs should be obtained to assess proximal lesions, despite considerations of radiation exposure.

Nevertheless, not all radiographically determined translucencies require treatment. This decision also must be made in accordance with the existing risk of caries. The rule holds that all treatment should be as minimal as possible. Small proximal lesions, for example, can be made accessible with elastic separators or brass wire separation. Composite restorations with the enamel-etching technique and amalgam restorations without extension can be considered. In every instance, this approach preserves the occlusal topography.

Sealing of pits and fissures

Immediately on eruption, the narrow tortuous fissures are colonized by microorganisms. At the same time, a fermentable substrate is pressed onto them and retained mechanically. Even with good oral hygiene, only the entrances to the fissures in the occlusal surfaces can be maintained plaque free (Galil and Gwinnett 1975). Deeper parts of the fissures remain unavoidably plaque retentive. Because of the thin, incomplete enamel layer in the occlusal region, such lesions that start in a fissure and quickly progress into the dentin near the pulp (Galil and Gwinnett 1975) (Figs 3-7a to 3-7c).

Depending on the condition of the fissure, the clinician has several choices (Heintze 1996b):

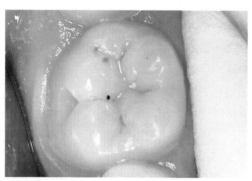

Fig 3-7a Initial appearance of the occlusal and buccal surface.

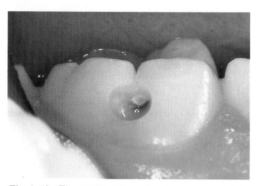

Fig 3-7b The carious invasion becomes visible after preparation of the buccal carious lesion.

Figs 3-7a to 3-7c Pit and fissure sealant is applied to the mandibular right first molar.

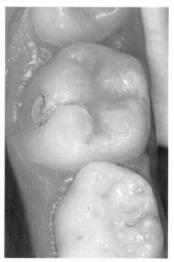

Fig 3-7c Fissure sealed with Delton Tinted. Buccal defect restored with amalgam (shown immediately after amalgam placement).

1. No treatment
2. Use of chlorhexidine against mutans streptococci
3. Application of fluoride for remineralization
4. Therapeutic fissure sealing
5. Conventional restoration

The type of treatment finally selected depends not only on the diagnosis but also on the age of the tooth and the individual's caries risk. Sealing of pits and fissures after tooth eruption can reduce the risk of caries for these surfaces. Even the progression of initial carious lesions can be stopped (Handelman et al 1985,

Mertz-Fairhurst et al 1986); therefore, questionable or early carious lesions should be sealed. If pits and fissures are sealed shortly after eruption, this ecosystem of mutans streptococci is separated from that of the remainder of the oral cavity. Removal of the microbes is not necessary, because they are enclosed and separated from any additional substrate (Going et al 1978, Weerheijm et al 1992).

The excellent caries-protective effect of fissure sealants has been substantiated in many studies. The longitudinal study of longest duration lasted more than 15 years (Simonsen 1991). Although only 27.6% of the surfaces retained the sealant after 1 year, 74% of the sealed surfaces

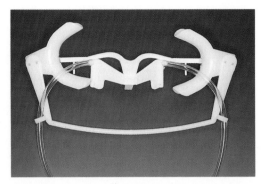

Fig 3-8a The Dry Field System is a combination of lip, cheek, and tongue retractors with an integrated saliva ejector for optimal relative isolation of tooth surfaces.

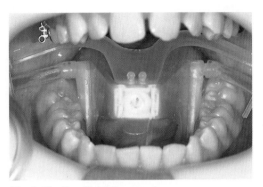

Fig 3-8b Dry Field System in use.

remained free of caries after 15 years. In the control group, in contrast, 82.8% of the surfaces were carious. Despite the small number of patients (24), it is fair to conclude that unsealed occlusal surfaces of first molars have a 7.5 times greater probability of becoming carious than do sealed surfaces.

The US National Institutes of Health, for that reason, expressly recommends the sealing of pits and fissures to reduce caries in the population significantly beyond that already achieved through fluorides and other measures (NIH 1984). Nevertheless, a recent survey revealed that only about 18% of US children have their teeth sealed (Selwitz et al 1996).

Use of rubber dam

Placement of a rubber dam before application of sealant to pits and fissures, while always desirable, should not be elevated to the status of dogma. Use of a rubber dam often is impossible because of the conical shape of a particular tooth. Early placement of sealant without a rubber dam, under conditions that are as dry as possible, is better than waiting for the possibility of placing rubber dam clamps (Heintze 1996a and 1996b). For instance, the Dry Field System (Figs 3-8a and 3-8b) is available for easy and successful preparation of a dry field. With the help of a good dental assistant, the practitioner can also achieve a satisfactorily dry field with suction, a saliva ejector, and cotton rolls (Paterson et al 1991).

Placement of sealant

Placement of sealant always should be delayed until the tooth surface to be treated has erupted completely. Moisture from the gingiva covering a partially erupted tooth can compromise the success of sealant application (Walker et al 1990).

According to Fejerskov (1995), prophylactic fissure sealing is problematic since the sealant is almost regularly lost. Primarily all efforts should be directed toward a reduction of cariogenic microorganisms. In contrast to prophylactic sealing, therapeutic sealing has a clear indication. Therapeutic sealing requires removal of existing caries and thus provides a better and larger etching pattern for subsequent adhesion (Le Bell and Forsten 1980, De Graene et al 1988).

Personal experience over the years leads us to recommend a transparent, tinted, resin composite material, Delton Tinted, for all forms of fissure sealing. Its advantages include simple, quick application (syringe application and self-curing) and good coverage of the prepared enamel. This positive evaluation has been confirmed in various studies (Houpt and Sheykholeslam 1978, Brooks et al 1979). In an in vitro thermocycling study in our dental school, Delton was found to be significantly superior to Helioseal (Loundos 1997). Significantly more marginal gaps and sealant fractures were found at the margins of Helioseal.

No secondary caries or total loss of sealant was found in a follow-up study of approximately 1200 therapeutic fissure sealings with Delton Tinted material. Small marginal gaps were found at palatal extensions of maxillary molars in a few instances; similar findings were observed in combined occlusal-buccal sealings of mandibular molars. The explanation for this lies in the shrinkage of the composite material. For that reason, sealants should not be placed on large surfaces or as multisurface applications.

Application of sealant

Application of a therapeutic sealing involves the following steps (Figs 3-9a to 3-9f):

1. *Providing isolation* (see Figs 3-8a and 3-8b). Isolation may be achieved with a rubber dam, cotton rolls, saliva ejector and suction, or the Dry Field System.

2. *Minimally invasive removal of caries.* The depth of the fissure is exposed through preparation with a small pointed fine-grained diamond bur. If any caries remains, it is excavated.

3. *Potential interferences between fluoridation and etching pattern.* A comparative study found no interference in the etching pattern from fluoride (Nordenvall et al 1980). For that reason, an application of fluoride before etching could be continued. Even high-dose varnish applications 24 hours before sealing have no effect on the etching pattern (Silverstone 1984).

   In a therapeutic fissure sealing, the preparation itself cleans and polishes the surface thoroughly (see Figs 3-9a and 3-9b). Preparatory cleaning with prophylaxis paste therefore is not required; however, if a prophylactic paste is used, the surface must be rinsed thoroughly. Paste particles that remain on the surface can disturb the etching process.

4. *Etching the enamel* (see Fig 3-9c). Etching the enamel surface with 30% to 40% phosphoric acid dissolves the enamel selectively, leading to the formation of voids in which the composite is retained. At the same time, marginal gaps are impeded.

   Etchants are available as liquids and as gels. The advantage of the gel is its high viscosity, which permits the gel to be placed more precisely. The advantage of the liquid, in contrast, lies in the fact that a less precise application guarantees etching of a larger surface. Broad etching prevents coverage of unetched enamel by composite, which could lead to marginal gaps and secondary caries.

   The practitioner should not hold rigidly to an etching time of 60 seconds, because there is no scientific

Figs 3-9a to 3-9f Clinical procedure for therapeutic fissure sealing.

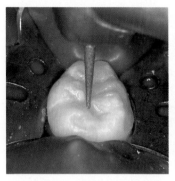

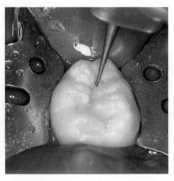

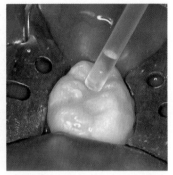

Fig 3-9a Preparation of the fissure with a fine-grained diamond.

Fig 3-9b Excavation of carious dentin.

Fig 3-9c Etching of the enamel around the fissure.

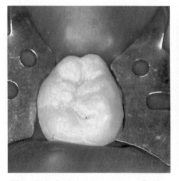

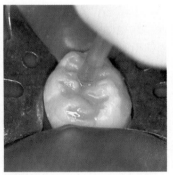

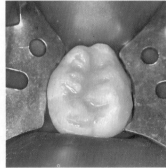

Fig 3-9d Appearance of the etched enamel regions.

Fig 3-9e Application of the tinted sealant with a special applicator.

Fig 3-9f Appearance after completion of sealing.

evidence for it; etching for 15 seconds suffices in a young dentition. An in vivo study found no difference in adhesive force after etching times of 15 and 60 seconds (Barkmeier et al 1986). Furthermore, the duration of the entire process is shortened by a reduced etching time.

5. *Rinsing the etched enamel.* Rinsing removes the dissolved enamel products that would otherwise impair adhesion. Studies have shown that a

rinsing period of 15 to 20 seconds is sufficient (Schulein et al 1986). The previously recommended 60-second spray does not lead to a better etching pattern; on the contrary, it leads to injury to the surface and flattening of the etching pattern (Mixson et al 1988).

6. *Drying the etched area.* Oil-free air is used to dry the tooth. A well-etched enamel surface has an opaque appearance after drying (see Fig 3-9d).

The period between drying of the surface and application of the sealant is the critical time in the sealing process, because no moisture must be permitted to reach the etched area. If saliva touches the etched surface, the spaces produced by etching are filled with salivary proteins, which cannot be removed by rinsing. Therefore, if saliva contaminates the surface, fresh etchant must be applied; a 5-second application suffices.

7. *Applying and polymerizing the sealant* (see Figs 3-9e and 3-9f). Two-component systems, eg, Delton Tinted, which polymerize through chemical means, and light-curing systems, eg, Helioseal, are available commercially. Since air bubbles destroy the integrity of the sealant, they must be avoided during mixing and application. If air bubbles nevertheless occur, they must be removed. Special advantages of Delton Tinted include low viscosity, low surface tension, and simple, quick application. A disadvantage of the light-curing sealants is their need for an additional step (light exposure) following application.

8. *Removing excess sealant and providing fluoridation.* Thin layers of excess sealant do not polymerize because of oxygen inhibition and therefore are easily removed with a cotton pledget soaked in a fluoride solution. This also ensures fluoridation of the etched but not sealed enamel surface, promoting remineralization.

9. *Checking the margins and the occlusion.* The margins are checked with an explorer and finished with a composite finisher if necessary. As a rule, the occlusion is not disturbed by sealant ap-

plication, but it should be checked nonetheless (Figs 3-10a and 3-10b).

10. *Checking the sealant 3 months after application.* Studies have shown that sealings undergo their most critical phase in the first several months after application. If examination reveals loss of sealant or a marginal gap, the sealant should be reapplied.

Although therapeutic sealing is invasive and requires an additional step, ie, the preparation, it has some advantages:

1. Sealant placement can be delayed. Only high-risk fissures with initial lesions are sealed; overtreatment is avoided.

2. Opening of the fissure permits better estimation of the demineralization and removal of existing caries.

3. The preparation process obviates the need for cleaning of the enamel surface.

4. The preparation process removes the superficial aprismatic enamel, thus improving the subsequent etching pattern.

Specific tooth surfaces can be treated with a sealing even while the teeth are banded (Fig 3-11).

Sealants that release fluoride (Fluoroshield, Helioseal-F) were developed to combine the effect of the mechanical closure of fissures with the remineralizing effect of fluoride. As is true in the case of bracket adhesives, the fluoride does not significantly decrease the adhesion of the sealant (Jensen et al 1990). However, fluoride is released very quickly after placement, which then questions the caries-inhibitory effect. If the sealing of a fissure is complete, fluoride release to prevent secondary caries is unnecessary.

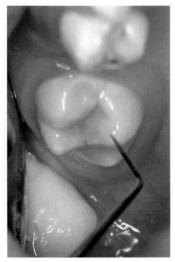

Fig 3-10a The margins of the sealant are checked with an explorer.

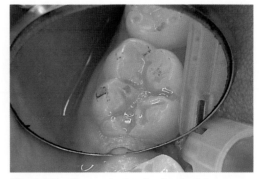

Fig 3-10b The occlusion is checked to ensure that the sealant does not interfere with maximum intercuspation.

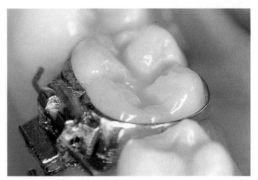

Fig 3-11 Fissure sealant has been placed on the tooth after banding.

Glass-ionomer cement sealant

The advantage of using glass-ionomer cements as sealants are their adherence to dentin and enamel, which precludes the need for etching. Also, this chemical bonding process is very desirable and ensures that fluoride ions that act cariostatically are released over a long period.

A glass-ionomer cement (Fuji III) and two resin composite sealants (Delton and Concise) were compared in a 5-year study

(Mejàre and Mjör 1990). Although almost 100% of the glass-ionomer cement seals showed some loss of sealant clinically after 5 years (in contrast to only 10% of the composite seals), not a single fissure that had been sealed with glass-ionomer cement was associated with secondary caries; such lesions were found in 5% of the fissures that had been treated with composite sealants. The authors ascribe their results to the fact that remnants of the glass-ionomer cement remained in the fissures, as demonstrated electron microscopically by a replication technique. These results should not, however, be interpreted as an unreserved recommendation for glass-ionomer cements as sealants, particularly because the findings have not been confirmed. A recently published review of the literature indicated that retention for resin-based sealants is better than for glass-ionomer sealants, but differences in caries prevention remain the same (Simonsen 1996). Further research should concentrate on the role of fluoride release of sealant materials for caries inhibition.

DIETARY COUNSELING

The relationship between amount and frequency of sucrose intake and the development of caries is unchallenged. Frequent sugar consumption promotes the growth of cariogenic organisms significantly and thus increases the risk of caries. Therefore it is necessary to stress, during dietary counseling, that between-meal snacks and hidden sugar be avoided. Four to six portions of sweets a day do not generally pose a danger.

It is desirable, before the beginning of any orthodontic treatment, to determine the dietary habits of a given patient. Exact establishment of nutritional habits is inordinately complex and hardly subject to objective analysis. The following are among the more commonly used methods:

1. The dietary interview. The dentist or the dental hygienist reviews the patient's nutritional habits with the aid of a questionnaire. This sort of interview is better suited for the purpose than having the unsupervised patient complete the form (Schröder et al 1981). In the process, an ordinary day is simulated and the average frequency of intake of specific nutritional components is noted. Special care is given to sweet between-meal snacks. Points are ascribed to each answer and a total point count is noted (Nizel 1981).

2. The 24-hour recall. The patient is asked to recall everything he or she has consumed in the previous 24 hours (Martinsson 1972).

3. The nutritional protocol. The patient records everything he or she eats and drinks over a 3- or 7-day period (Johnsen et al 1980).

These methods share the disadvantage that the subjects—including children and adolescents—all have at least a subconscious idea of the significance of sugar consumption on the development of caries. That knowledge may encourage incorrect statements so that certain caries-promoting dietary habits are denied.

Assessment of dietary habits. The evaluation of the cariogenicity of specific foods depends less on the absolute content of sucrose than on the average sucrose clearing time, ie, how high is the salivary glucose concentration and how quickly is it lowered? The caries potential index, developed by Lundqvist (1952) takes both sucrose content and clearance time into consideration. The cariogenicity of certain foods is listed in Table 3-1.

It is important to ascertain which cariogenic foods are consumed as snacks and the frequency of their consumption. Sweet snacks and drinks between meals are the greatest danger to dental health, even when, as in the case of drinks, clearance is rapid and therefore the danger should be lower.

Table 3-1 Sucrose content, clearance time, and caries potentiality index of selected foods

Food	Absolute sucrose content (%)	Mean sucrose clearance time (min)	Caries potentiality index
Caramel	64.0	5.00	27
Honey + bread	19.0	7.50	24
Chocolate	47.5	6.25	21
Honey	72.8	5.00	18
Sweet roll	9.0	5.00	18
Cake	30.0	2.50	13
White bread	12.3	4.00	13
Marmalade	65.3	3.50	10
Ice cream	2.4	2.50	9
White bread + butter	2.3	2.00	7
Rye bread + butter	2.3	2.00	7
Lemonade	9.3	0.75	2
Fruit juice	11.5	1.00	3
Milk	3.8	2.00	6
Apple	7.5	1.00	5
Orange	6.5	1.00	3

From Lundqvist 1952.

If a discrepancy exists between the patient's statements and the clinical condition, the truth can be established with a lactobacilli test, because the number of lactobacilli present is related closely to the amount of carbohydrate consumed. A lactobacilli test serves as an indicator of sugar consumption. The presence of more than 1 million colony-forming units per milliliter of saliva reflects high sugar intake with certainty. However, this test demonstrates not only the lactobacilli present as a consequence of consumption of carbohydrate, but also those present in natural and artificial retention niches (carious lesions, restorations with marginal gaps or overhangs, and fixed orthodontic appliances) (Crossner and Hagberg 1977). This places the following limits on the test:

1. The first lactobacilli test should be done before orthodontic treatment is initiated.

2. All open carious lesions (including those in the primary dentition) should be restored, at least provisionally, and inadequate restorations should be replaced.

3. The test should be repeated to evaluate preventive measures and their effect.

Useful conversion of the newly gained, semireliable understanding of the patient's carbohydrate consumption may be difficult. Repeated urging that the patient eat tooth-friendly foods is often useless, particularly if much dietary change would be required. Nonetheless, the dentist and the dental hygienist must make every effort to explain the problems associated with the patient's diet. Small changes and adjustments are accepted more readily and maintained over longer periods by the patient than are radical cures. Only in the presence of nursing bottle caries must the clinician rigorously insist on change and instruct the parent to take the bottle away from the child immediately.

That repeated promotion of low-carbohydrate foods is not without success is demonstrated by statistics from Scandinavia. In Sweden, Norway, and Finland, only 8%, 16% and 21% of 11-year-olds,

respectively, eat between-meal sweets every day (Honkala et al 1990). The "sugar clock," broadly distributed in Scandinavia, can be a useful aid in motivation (Fig 3-12) (Ainamo 1980). It depicts a readily understandable version of the so-called Stephan curve. More than 50 years ago, Stephan (1944) examined the effect of sucrose intake on plaque. The drop in pH in the plaque can last up to 30 minutes after sucrose intake. Such pH diagrams are difficult for the patient to understand. Thus, the sugar clock is an aid in explaining the relation between "acid attack" and "caries defeat." The patient marks his or her sugar intake at half-hour intervals on an outline of a clock face with a red marker. The more frequently sugar is consumed, the more vividly is the duration of acid attack depicted on the clock face. In this way, the patient has an immediate visual depiction of his or her misdeeds with sugar.

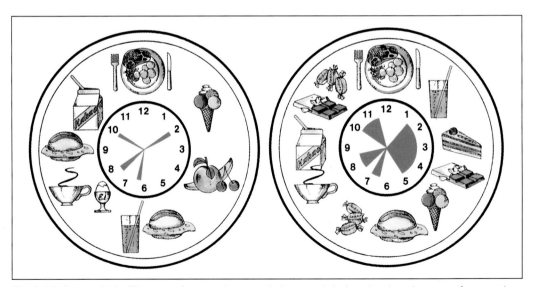

Fig 3-12 Sugar clock. The more frequently sugar is ingested during the day, the more frequently a red shade appears on the face of the clock.

Dietary guidelines for patients

Beyond such measures, patients must be motivated to use less sugar in the preparation of their foods. Sugar is not a food; it is a spice and should be used accordingly. It would be desirable if the food industry would reduce the sugar content of its products or remove it entirely from some foods. For all patients, but particularly for children, sugar hidden in foods in which its presence is unsuspected is especially dangerous. Examples include mustard, sausage, tomato ketchup, cough drops, sialagogues, and all syrups, including those that serve as "packing material" for drugs intended for use in children.

If the patient is unable to give up products containing sugar, he or she must at least be encouraged to consume them strategically. In effect, that means consumption at mealtime and not between meals. In addition, "tooth-friendly" products that substitute xylitol, sorbitol, or aspartame for sucrose can be an alternative.

Worthy of recommendation in this regard is the use of sugarless chewing gum. Chewing leads to increased salivary flow, which increases the buffer capacity and the saturation of saliva with ions that promote remineralization (Manning and Edgar 1992). Although chewing gum that contains sugar also increases salivary flow, some studies have found it to be caries promoting (review Edgar and Geddes 1990). Longitudinal studies over the past 20 years indicate that daily chewing of xylitol-based chewing gum can lead to 30% to 85% caries reduction. In some instances, active lesions in children were brought to a halt (Makinen 1993).

Home-Care Measures for Reducing Oral Bacteria

4

It may be stating the obvious to note that home oral hygiene is important. Every cleaning technique is appropriate, to the extent that it removes microbial plaque. Another fundamental bit of wisdom relates to the importance of instructing and motivating patients and their parents regularly. The posterior teeth (especially lingually in the mandible and buccally in the maxilla) are the problem zones.

The uppermost goal of all efforts in this connection is the development of the patient's sensitivity to the cleanliness of his or her teeth. For example, the patient should be taught to feel deposits on the teeth with the tongue. Although children should be taught to clean their teeth themselves as early as possible, it remains the responsibility of the parents to check the results of the cleaning and to complete the process if necessary.

ASSESSMENT OF ORAL HYGIENE

Disclosing agents

Use of disclosing agents to check thoroughness of cleaning is in order. A variety of disclosing materials are available.

Erythrosin was the first dye to be used in dentistry for this purpose. Brilliant blue, malachite green, and fluorescein also are used; the last becomes visible in ultraviolet light.

Erythrosin preferably dyes "fresh" plaque; older plaque is disclosed better with fluorescein and brilliant blue. Complex dye systems such as 2-Tone, which contains fluorescein and brilliant blue, permit differentiation between newly formed and older plaque (Block et al 1972) (Fig 4-1). Plaque that has been present for 3 days or more has more cariogenic (and periodontopathic) potential than 1- or 2-day-old plaque, because older plaque is more structured and contains more acid-forming organisms. In practice, however, the patient must be motivated to remove all plaque.

An erythrosin solution is a suitable and inexpensive disclosing material for use in the dental office and at home. An inexpensive solution prepared by a pharmacist (5% erythrosin with one drop of oil of anise per 5 mL) is as effective as commercially available solutions (Kieser and Wade 1976) (Figs 4-2a and 4-2b). It is best to apply the erythrosin solution with a cotton-tipped applicator. To protect the lips from discoloration, a light layer of creme (eg, petroleum jelly) may be applied beforehand.

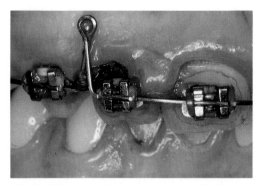

Fig 4-1 Plaque has been disclosed with 2-Tone. Old plaque appears dark blue (especially gingivally), while fresh plaque is reddish.

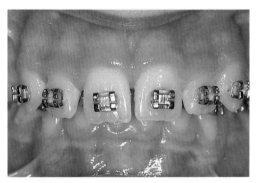

Fig 4-2a Before application of disclosing solution, plaque is barely visible.

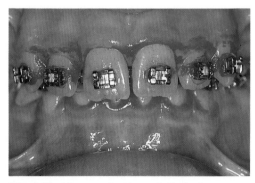

Fig 4-2b After application of disclosing material, deposits are evident, particularly in the proximal spaces and in the "shadow" of the archwires, ie, mesial and distal to the brackets. One-time use of a disclosing agent motivates patients very little; the effect is much better when the procedure shown in Fig 4-3 is used.

As an aid to motivation and to improve the patient's understanding of the relationship between oral hygiene and plaque formation, it is beneficial to clean one anterior tooth professionally before use of a disclosing solution. When the erythrosin solution has been applied to all the teeth, only that tooth will be free of coloring agent (Fig 4-3). However, only a thorough discussion makes the patient aware of the relationship between plaque and oral hygiene, and that knowledge is the decisive prerequisite for effective oral hygiene (Kipioti et al 1984).

Esthetic problems may arise in patients with fixed appliances. All disclosing agents except fluorescein, no matter the manufacturer, discolor elastics (Fig 4-4). Our own experience has indicated that adhesive resin is only very weakly dyed. If the discoloration disturbs the patient excessively, or he or she does not want to change the elastics frequently, only fluorescein is suitable as the disclosing medium.

Ceramic brackets pose another problem. The dye penetrates microscopically small tears and irregularities, giving the bracket a permanent red, blue, or green cast. Only fluorescein should be used by patients with ceramic brackets.

Over the past several years, plaque-disclosing agents have been said to be carcinogenic. Fuchsin, for example, was banned many years ago. Because it was found to be weakly mutagenic in bacterial studies (van de Rijke 1991), erythrosin was forbidden by the US Food and Drug Administration several years ago; erythrosin may elicit an allergy in sensitive persons (FAO/WHO 1975). If instead natural liquids (eg, elderberry) are used as an alternative, the staining contrast is weaker.

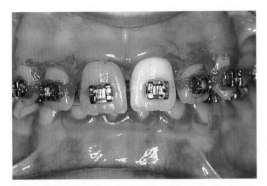

Fig 4-3 Professional cleaning of a single tooth before use of a disclosing solution can be a useful aid to motivation.

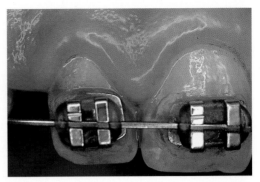

Fig 4-4 The previously colorless rubber ligatures have been discolored irreversibly by malachite green.

Oral hygiene indices

It is desirable to determine a plaque and/or gingival index to obtain current information about the present state of the patient's oral hygiene and the gingiva. The O'Leary hygiene index (O'Leary et al 1972) is an appropriate plaque index; the Ainamo (Ainamo and Bay 1975) gingival bleeding index (GBI) is suitable as a gingival index (see chapter 2). Both indices are practical and require only a yes or no decision. The GBI should be determined before any disclosing medium is applied.

All teeth must be stained with a liquid disclosing solution to determine the numerical value of O'Leary's hygiene index. It is best to apply the disclosing solution with a cotton pledget or a cotton-tipped applicator. The patient is asked to rinse, so that only the tooth surfaces to which plaque adheres remain stained. The presence or absence of plaque is recorded. The points of measurement are identical to those used for the GBI: facial, oral, mesioproximal, and distoproximal. A quotient is determined so that the percentage of teeth affected can be calculated. An ex-

ample of the plaque index determination is found in Fig 4-5.

Other indices, such as the Lange approximal plaque index, the Quigley-Hein index, the Silness and Löe plaque index, the Saxer and Mühlemann papillary bleeding index, the oral hygiene index, or the sulcus bleeding index, can be used as well. In general, however, these indices appear too unspecific for use in individuals or complicate the diagnosis because their values are expressed in stages. At the same time, these indices have the inherent danger of subjective underestimation or overestimation, particularly when they are determined by several observers for the same patient.

In 1989 Declerk and coworkers developed a device to analyze the occurrence of plaque automatically, to improve quantification of the colored tooth surfaces and to reduce subjective deviation in the estimation of indices.

Ortho-plaque index

Large portions of the buccal surfaces (and sometimes the lingual surfaces as well) are covered by adhesive attachments in pa-

$$\frac{\text{Number of stained sites}}{\text{Total number of sites}} \times 100 = \% \text{ plaque affected}$$

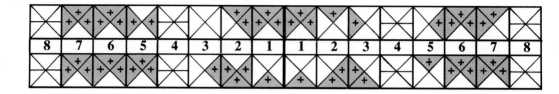

$$\frac{49}{96} \times 100 = 51\% \text{ plaque affected}$$

Fig 4-5 Example of the O'Leary hygiene (or plaque) index. All tooth surfaces are treated with a disclosing material. The presence of stain is recorded for four sites: facial, lingual, mesioproximal, and distoproximal. Sites with plaque are counted. All premolars have been extracted in the present example, reducing the number of sites measured.

tients with fixed appliances. Regions cervical to the bracket base and those mesial and distal to the arch wire are the most critical zones of plaque formation (Fig 4-6). Therefore it is desirable to evaluate these zones separately for a plaque index. For this purpose we developed the ortho-plaque index.

The points of measurement for this index are cervical, mesial or distal, and coronal to the bracket (Figs 4-7a and 4-7b). As with the O'Leary index, a yes or no decision is recorded: Is plaque present at the site of measurement? This index does not differentiate between mesial and distal surfaces; if plaque is found in one of these regions, the result is positive.

So that a quick determination can be made during routine appointments, and to motivate the patient for oral hygiene, the findings are weighted in accordance with their accessibility to tooth-cleaning: occlusal = 1, easily accessible; cervical = 2, accessible with some difficulty; and under the orthodontic archwire = 3, poorly accessible (see Fig 4-6).

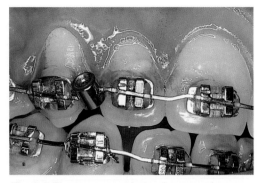

Fig 4-6 Plaque accumulation is extensive, particularly mesial and distal to the brackets.

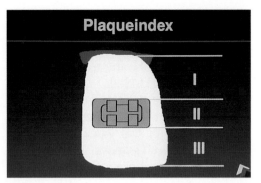

Fig 4-7a Ortho-plaque index (OPI). First, all buccal surfaces of bonded teeth are stained with a disclosing agent. Each tooth has three sites for measurement: cervical (I), the region of the "shadow" of the archwire, mesial and distal to the bracket (II = central), and coronal to the bracket (III = occlusal).

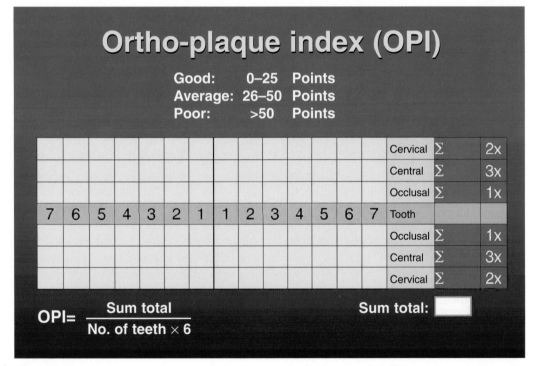

Ortho-plaque index (OPI)

Good: 0–25 Points
Average: 26–50 Points
Poor: >50   Points

															Cervical Σ	2x
															Central Σ	3x
															Occlusal Σ	1x
7	6	5	4	3	2	1	1	2	3	4	5	6	7		Tooth	
															Occlusal Σ	1x
															Central Σ	3x
															Cervical Σ	2x

$$OPI = \frac{Sum\ total}{No.\ of\ teeth \times 6}$$

Sum total: ☐

Fig 4-7b The presence or absence of plaque at each site is recorded. The number of sites with plaque is added, and these totals are multiplied by factors: 1 for the coronal, 2 for the cervical, and 3 for the archwire section of a given tooth. The OPI is the sum of the resulting numbers divided by number of teeth present x 6 x 100^{-1}.

To establish the presence of plaque as a percentage, the number of sites affected by plaque is multiplied by the weighting factor and divided by the total number of sites present. Banded teeth are not counted, nor are third molars in a complete dentition; the latter rarely are banded. Users of this index can quickly evaluate the oral hygiene of a patient wearing a fixed appliance, according to the following schedule: 0% to 30% represents good oral hygiene; 30% to 50% represents fair oral hygiene; more than 50% represents poor oral hygiene.

To date, subjective experience with this index has been positive. Scientific evaluation, including comparison with other indices, remains to be completed.

CLEANING OF FIXED APPLIANCES

All efforts of the dental team must be supported and supplemented by home care. Professional oral hygiene measures alone cannot reduce the cariogenicity and periodontal pathogenicity of deposits on the teeth, because recolonization with bacteria occurs immediately after each such procedure. Without daily oral hygiene by the patients, no positive results should be anticipated.

Toothbrush design

The toothbrush to be used should have a short head to reach all regions of the teeth. Additional characteristics of a toothbrush worth recommending include a straight brush field; rounded, multitufted bristles; and, for smaller children, a large handle. The toothbrush should be discarded when the first sign of bending appears on the bristles; this may happen in 4 to 8 weeks.

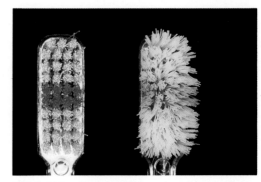

Fig 4-8 The Oral-B Indicator is said to indicate need for replacement through disappearance of the blue-colored central section. The brush on the right was used twice daily for 6 weeks before the central rows of bristles began to fade. However, two weeks earlier the outer bristles had begun to bend, so that the brush no longer was useful.

A toothbrush that indicates the time for replacement using color was introduced some time ago (Oral-B Indicator). The central rows of bristles are treated with a dye that disappears after a certain time of use. The outer rows of bristles, however, frequently show signs of bending long before that occurs, especially if the brush is used with much pressure. Therefore, the additional usefulness of this toothbrush is questionable (Fig 4-8).

Patients with gingival recession or wedge-shaped defects must be especially careful in their choice of toothbrushes and use only an extremely soft variety. Besides other factors, the toothpaste (its abrasivity and grinding and polishing agents) plays an important role, as do the type and frequency of toothbrushing.

Cleaning technique

A patient with fixed appliances must devote special attention to the care of his or her teeth because cleaning is impeded. While the cervical surfaces pose a problem in banded teeth, also the surfaces mesial and distal to the adhesive surfaces—those in the "shadow" of the archwire—pose difficulties in teeth with brackets. These surfaces are poorly accessible to the bristles of any toothbrush. Severe plaque formation and subsequent demineralization may result in these regions (Fig 4-9).

Toothbrush manufacturers market special brushes with shortened bristles in the center of the brush head to reach these poorly accessible areas better. However, these special brushes provide no signifi-

cant advantage over conventional brushes, given proper brushing technique and application of sufficient force to the head of the conventional brush (Hotz et al 1984, Williams et al 1987).

Proper brushing technique primarily means separate brushing of the tooth surfaces lying occlusal and cervical to the arch wire. Patients with fixed appliances should apply more force than usual when using their brush. An increase in applied force from 0.6 to 5.0 N led to a 47% decrease in plaque deposition in patients with fixed appliances (White et al 1989).

Lingually or palatally placed retentive elements make cleaning particularly difficult, because the lingual surfaces are neglected in general, with both, the toothbrush (Rugg-Gunn et al 1979) and dental floss (Ong 1990). This neglect can lead quickly to gingival hyperplasia around lingual brackets or other attachments (Gorman et al 1983), as is observed frequently, particularly in the region of the anterior teeth (Figs 4-10a and 4-10b).

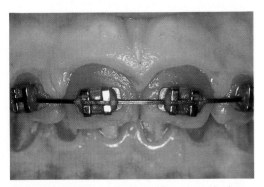

Fig 4-9 Cervical tooth surfaces and those under archwires are poorly accessible to cleaning and therefore are exposed to heavy deposits (stained here with erythrosin).

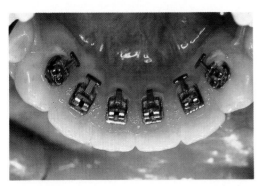

Fig 4-10a Gingival hyperplasia is evident around the mandibular anterior teeth, which have lingually bonded brackets. The pseudopockets pose additional retention sites for plaque, initiating a vicious cycle of more gingival hyperplasia.

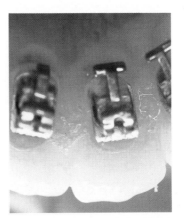

Fig 4-10b Close-up of a section of Fig 4-10a shows the extent of gingival hyperplasia. The hyperplastic papillae almost reach the incisal level of the brackets.

These pseudopockets form an additional retention area for plaque and can accelerate lingual demineralization.

The so-called scrub technique (horizontal back and forth movement) has been recommended for patients with fixed appliances (Clark 1976, Zachrisson 1976). Standardized examinations with an in vitro model, however, showed the modified Bass technique (rotation technique) to be superior to the scrub method for patients

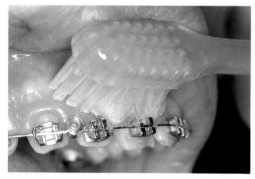

Fig 4-11a The toothbrush is positioned for cleaning the gingival areas.

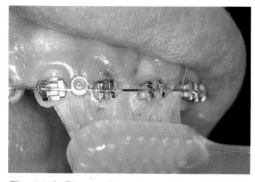

Fig 4-11b The toothbrush must be turned toward the occlusal surface or the incisal edge to clean the coronal tooth surfaces.

with fixed appliances (Hotz et al 1984). A modified Bass technique (small, circular shaking motions, while the brush is held at a 45-degree angle to tooth axis) was also shown to be superior to the roll technique (rotating motions from the sulcus to the occlusal surface) in a clinical study, because plaque removal was better on smooth surfaces (Kremers et al 1983). Because many patients place the toothbrush too far coronally, the gingival sectors are neglected routinely, leading to increased plaque formation and subsequent gingivitis. All patients therefore must be instructed to clean the tooth surfaces cervical to the brackets and bands (Clark 1976) (Figs 4-11a and 4-11b).

A toothbrush alone is not enough to clean dental arches with bonded or banded appliances. Daily use of Superfloss and interdental brushes is recommended. Superfloss is stiffened and narrowed at one end so that insertion behind or below the arch wire is eased. The brackets can thus be cleaned well with the soft portion, but not the enamel mesial and distal to the bracket bases themselves, because the tuftlike thicker portion of the floss is too soft (Figs 4-12a and 4-12b; 4-13a and 4-13b).

Interdental brushes that have stiff handles so that they are not bent down are more suitable for these regions (Figs 4-14a to 4-14c). Furthermore, such brushes should have only rounded bristles so that the gingiva is not harmed. Among 14 interdental brushes examined, however, none fulfilled these requirements completely (Reiter and Wetzel 1991). Also with single-tufted brushes, the tooth surfaces proximal to the brackets and under the bands may be cleaned sufficiently (Figs 4-15a to 4-15c).

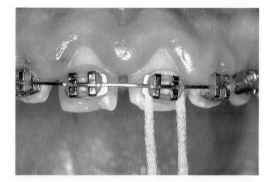

Fig 4-12a Dental floss with a soft portion (Superfloss) reaches the surfaces around the brackets poorly.

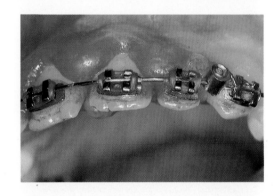

Fig 4-12b After five passes with Superfloss, plaque remains.

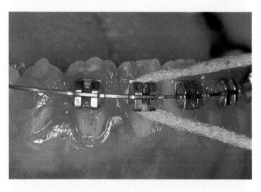

Fig 4-13a The plaque has been dyed before the use of Superfloss.

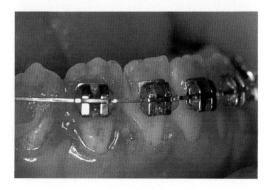

Fig 4-13b Traces of plaque remain around the bracket base.

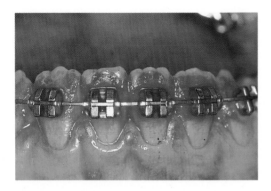

Figs 4-14a to 4-14c Efficient plaque removal around the lateral bracket bases is possible with an interdental brush.

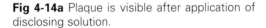

Fig 4-14a Plaque is visible after application of disclosing solution.

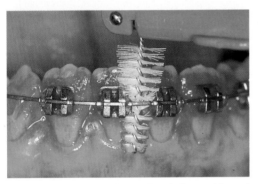

Fig 4-14b The interdental brush is positioned for use.

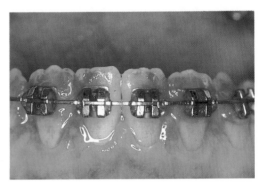

Fig 4-14c The removal of plaque is obvious following passes of the brush between the brackets.

Interdental brushes have the advantage of removing subgingival plaque, to a depth of 2.0 to 2.5 mm (Waerhaug 1976). Thus, even bands placed below the gingival margin can be freed from plaque. However, it is practically impossible to reach into the interdental space of children with even the smallest interdental brushes (Fig 4-16). Dental floss or Superfloss is more suitable in these regions.

It is not certain that Superfloss removes plaque from the proximal surfaces better than ordinary floss. A study by Abelson et al (1981) indicated Superfloss to be superior to waxed floss; in other studies, no significant differences, in terms of the plaque index, were found between the two types (Bergenholtz and Brithon 1980, Ong 1990). The volume of the soft part of Superfloss is too large for the papillae of children and adolescents.

Nonetheless, this special dental floss, because of its stiffened end, offers the sole means of being threaded interdentally under the archwire of fixed appliances (Figs 4-17a and 4-17b). Superfloss also has the ability, as a result of its soft component, to reach subgingival band margins to remove plaque there (Figs 4-18a and 4-18b).

Figs 4-15a to 4-15c Tooth surfaces proximal to the brackets can be cleaned efficiently with a single-tufted brush (Elmex, with conically arranged, rounded synthetic bristles).

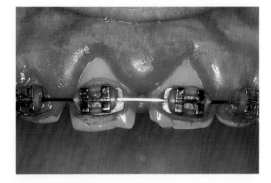

Fig 4-15a Plaque has been disclosed before brushing.

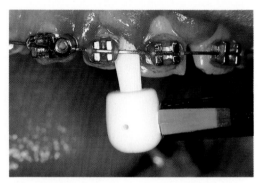

Fig 4-15b The brush is used between the central and lateral incisors.

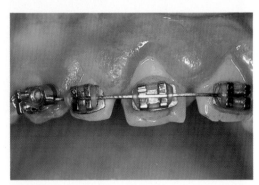

Fig 4-15c The elimination of plaque is nearly complete.

Fig 4-16 An interdental brush can be used to clean proximal surfaces only in adults (and in temporary gaps during treatment).

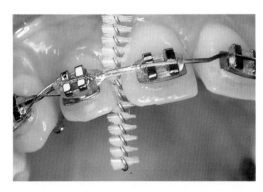

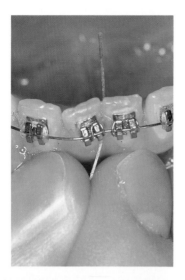

Fig 4-17a The stiffened end of a piece of Superfloss is inserted under the archwire. If sufficient space exists gingivally between two teeth, Superfloss can be threaded lingually. Otherwise, it must be pushed over the contact point.

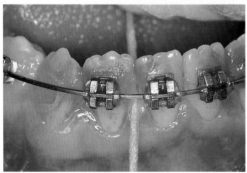

Fig 4-17b The teeth can be cleaned well with the inserted floss.

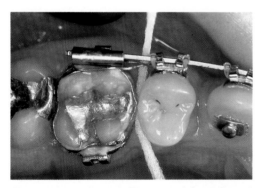
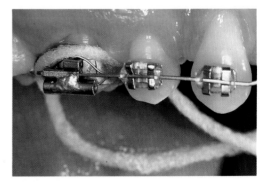

Figs 4-18a and 4-18b The use of Superfloss is particularly practical with bands, because the soft portion of the floss can reach subgingival margins.

Other cleaning aids, such as wooden or plastic toothpicks, are poorly suited to remove plaque safely (Bergenholtz and Brithon 1980); they roughen the dental enamel and easily traumatize the interdental papillae (Smith et al 1986).

Cleaning technique for proximal spaces

The positive effect of dental floss in the prevention of proximal caries is undisputed. Cleansing of the interdental spaces is also important from the point of view of periodontal health (Löe and Morrison, 1986). Studies have shown that gingivitis does not begin lingually or buccally, but always in the interdental space. In patients with periodontitis, as a rule, proximal probing depths are significantly greater than the buccal and, especially, the facial probing depths. Optimal plaque removal is attained only when dental floss is used regularly and thoroughly at least every 2 or 3 days. Brief flossing at shorter intervals has no effect.

If the patient experiences difficulties with conventional flossing, the dentist may suggest two alternatives:

1. A 12-inch piece of dental floss, knotted in the form of a sling, to avoid the need to wrap the floss around a finger (Fig 4-19)
2. A floss holder

The type of dental floss used, waxed or unwaxed, is of little consequence in plaque removal, although waxed floss is perceived to be more pleasant by most patients, because it tends to shred less and does not traumatize the papillae as much. Extra-wide-tooth-cleaning floss (Oral-B dental tape) simplifies plaque removal even more. Colgate provides a dental floss made of Gore-Tex fibers (Glide) that has

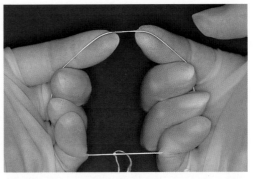

Fig 4-19 The requirement to clean every proximal space is fulfilled most easily if the ends of a piece of dental floss approximately 30 cm in length are knotted together. A part of the resulting loop, stretched between two fingers, is placed in the proximal spaces and moved about.

good gliding properties. It is extremely thin and tear-resistant and does not shred. Whether this material has clinical advantages and gains greater patient acceptance remains to be seen.

A recently introduced electric device for interdental cleaning (Interclean), which uses a rotating plastic filament, proved to be as efficient as dental flossing in young adults and may enhance patient compliance for interdental cleaning (Gordon et al 1996).

A new piece of dental floss should be used for each interdental space to avoid transfer of microorganisms between sites (Svanberg and Loesche 1978). Insertion of dental floss amounts to an "ecological catastrophe" for cariogenic bacteria because the structural organization of the plaque is destroyed; however, the number of organisms is reduced only insignificantly (Chaet and Wei 1977). Occasional cleaning of the interdental spaces with dental floss has no effect at all on the number of *Streptococcus mutans* in the plaque (Frandsen 1986).

All types of dental floss tear the junctional epithelium of healthy interdental papillae at the tooth surfaces; its regeneration generally requires 2 weeks. No irreparable damage need be anticipated. Patients, however, should be informed that it is not necessary to force the dental floss under the gingival margin of a healthy papilla, because no plaque exists there.

Interdental brushes are more effective and easier to use than dental floss when the interdental spaces are open as a result of periodontitis. All dental restorations must be designed so that interdental brushes can be used appropriately.

Cleaning technique for areas of recession and wedge-shaped defects

If recession is present, the patient should be trained in the Stillman brushing technique, which is a vertical-rotational brushing method. The brush is moved from the gingiva to the tooth, ie, from red to white. Initially, the brush is placed on the gingiva at an angle of approximately 45 degrees to the long axis of a tooth; the brush is turned around its long axis as it courses over the tooth surface. This motion is repeated at the same site 5 to 10 times. If the patient follows this procedure carefully, and if his or her oral hygiene is generally satisfactory, the progress of the recession ordinarily is halted.

Severe recession may be an indication for mucogingival surgery. A free gingival graft is placed in the effort to impede progression of the recession.

If the above-mentioned brushing recommendations are not followed, and an improper (horizontal) brushing technique is used, loss of dental hard tissue may occur in addition to recession of the gingiva. Excessively frequent brushing of long duration with an abrasive dentifrice quickly abrades the cementum exposed by a gingival recession. If, in addition, the patient consumes a diet containing high levels of acid, the process is accelerated. Such acid-containing foods include apples, citrus fruits, liquids enriched with vitamin C, soft drinks, and fruit drops. The purely chemical dissolution of cervical tooth enamel is called *erosion*. As a rule, however, the mechanical (toothbrushing) and the chemical (acid) components work together.

To prevent further destruction, the affected patient should be given the following recommendations:

1. After eating fruit or other foods or drinks containing acid, do not brush the teeth immediately. Wait at least 1 hour to give saliva, its ions, and the ions of the enamel and dentin time for reprecipitation.

2. Do not scrub horizontally. Instead, use the modified Stillman technique with a rolling cleaning motion.

3. Neutralize harmful acids by drinking milk or a solution of sodium bicarbonate (1 tsp in a quarter cup of water).

4. Use normal toothbrushes with straight, multitufted bristles. Brushes with natural bristles and those designated as hard are particularly injurious.

5. Use fluoridated dentifrices with a neutral or alkaline pH.

6. Avoid dentifrices that are excessively abrasive.

Frequency of toothbrushing

Increasing the frequency of toothbrushing does not lead automatically to cleaner teeth, particularly because certain tooth surfaces, such as the proximal surfaces, as well as the pits and fissures, are not optimally accessible to the toothbrush. Other means, such as dental floss, are required for interdental spaces. In consequence, the frequency of toothbrushing alone cannot be used as a measure of the quality of oral hygiene. Therefore, patients must be trained and their brushing procedures must be checked regularly.

Optimal toothbrushing once daily would be sufficient for caries protection. Even a 2-day interval would suffice for avoidance of gingivitis (Lang et al 1973). Administration of fluoride two or three times daily is desirable, however, to support remineralization. For that reason, the recommendation to brush after every meal remains justified, always assuming that the dentifrice contains fluoride.

A plaque formation rate index of III or higher (see chapter 2) is an indication of the need for greater frequency of toothbrushing. Patients who have an index of III or more, together with a high concentration of mutans streptococci in their saliva, should be cautioned to brush their teeth at least twice daily, mornings and evenings. The best time to brush is before meals, because preliminary effective plaque removal makes a decrease in pH following food uptake practically impossible, even when the food is rich in sucrose (Axelsson 1990).

According to Axelsson (1990), all oral hygiene measures should be need related. Thus, for example, cleaning of palatal surfaces is practically unnecessary, because these surfaces have an extremely low rate of plaque formation, ascribed to the cleaning effect of the constant coursing of the tongue over these surfaces. In contrast, special attention must be given to the linguoproximal surfaces of the mandibular molars (Fig 4-20) and the buccoproximal surfaces of the maxillary molars (Fig 4-21), because these have a great tendency for plaque formation. Despite these differences, it hardly seems advisable to suggest to patients that some surfaces may be ne-

glected. Rather, they should be encouraged to concentrate on the endangered surfaces.

In patients with fixed orthodontic appliances, it is important that the tooth surface with plaque-retentive elements be cleaned. Therefore, in practice, in patients with lingual appliances the palatal surfaces of the maxilla must be given attention, in addition to the lingual surfaces in the mandible, because the cleaning action of the tongue is limited.

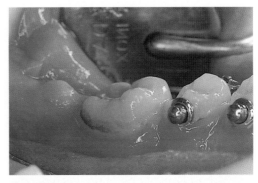

Fig 4-20 Special attention should be given to the linguoproximal surfaces of mandibular molars because much plaque accumulates in this region.

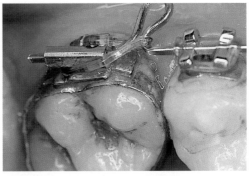

Fig 4-21 The buccoproximal surfaces of maxillary molars require special effort in cleaning because of increased plaque formation in this area.

ELECTRIC TOOTHBRUSHES

Conventional units

Manual brushing of the teeth is troublesome and time consuming for patients. Daily oral hygiene can become agony in the presence of fixed orthodontic appliances. Accordingly, it would be desirable to transfer this task in an optimal way to a machine. Most ordinary electric toothbrushes simply provide motorized replication of the movement of the hand-held toothbrush and are not superior to manual brushing techniques. These electric brushes offer a true alternative only for disabled patients. Yet, there are patients who cannot be motivated to intensive use of a manual toothbrush but who are nonetheless willing to use an electric toothbrush, which relieves them of some of the work.

Interplak

The Interplak unit features 10 rotating bristle bundles oscillating at 4,200 rpm. At the highest level of operation, each bundle changes its direction of rotation 46 times per second, according to the manufacturer. Use of dentifrices is not recommended with this device, because the abrasive components would quickly damage the sensitive mechanism of the brush head. For that reason, the manufacturer has developed a gel containing fluoride (Interplak tooth gel) without abrasive.

The Interplak device has been found to be better than the conventional manual brush method in clinical studies. In terms of plaque removal (Coontz 1985, Baab and Johnson 1989), and reduction of gingivitis (Killoy et al 1989), it is superior to conventional manual brushing. Proximal surfaces were reported to be 42.4% plaque free with Interplak but only 25.7% plaque free with a manual brush in a study

by Youngblood et al (1985). Another remarkable finding of this study was the greater penetration into the sulcus by the Interplak; 1.4 versus 0.7 mm with the manual toothbrush.

Despite these results, the problem zone of proximal surfaces remains. Supplemental use of dental floss or other aids is indispensable. An additional problem is that some patients perceive the Interplak brush as being too large and therefore often use it only once daily (Baab and Johnson 1989).

Rota-Dent

The Rota-Dent unit claims to clean the proximal surfaces optimally as well with three different brush heads, each of which includes 5000 filaments. The brush heads rotate at 800 to 1100 rpm (depending on the condition of the batteries) in a single direction.

In a 1-year study, the device was no more effective in plaque elimination and control of gingivitis in 20 periodontal patients than were conventional brushes, dental floss, and tooth picks in 20 control patients (Boyd et al 1989). Microbiologic findings were also similar (Murray et al 1989).

Plaque Remover

The heart of the plaque remover unit is a round brush head that rotates 70 degrees while oscillating at 2800 rpm. This frequency is said to provide the optimum relationship between cleaning effect and a pleasant cleaning feeling. The brush head consists of 27 circular bristle bundles with a total of 1500 rounded plastic bristles in a bowl-like arrangement.

A clinical study of 111 nonorthodontic patients over a 1-year period showed that no superiority of the device was found over a manual toothbrushing technique with respect to plaque removal (Ainamo et al 1997). In another study better plaque removal compared to a manual technique was only achieved when the investigators themselves did the cleaning or the subjects (dental students) were instructed in professional oral hygiene (van der Weijden et al 1993a).

When compared to Interplak, the Plaque Remover was equally effective after 15 seconds (van der Weijden et al 1993b). Two studies, however, revealed lower gingivitis indices for the Plaque Remover after 8 months and 12 months respectively when compared to a manual technique (van der Weijden et al 1994; Ainamo et al 1997).

Studies in orthodontic patients

Use of an electric toothbrush with rotating bristle heads may be particularly useful for patients with fixed orthodontic appliances because the tooth surfaces around the brackets and along the gingival band margins can be cleaned without much effort (Fig 4-22), as was made obvious in a clinical study. Fourteen orthodontic patients with plaque indices greater than 50%

cleaned their teeth on one side of the dental arch by hand with a toothbrush and the teeth on the other side with the Interplak device (Long and Killoy 1985). The Interplak was significantly better; about 84% of all mechanically cleaned teeth and only 66% of manually cleaned teeth were plaque free. Similarly positive was the decrease in signs of gingival inflammation in patients with fixed appliances who used this device (Yankell et al 1985; Wilcoxon et al 1991).

Results in patients with fixed orthodontic devices also are available for the Rota-Dent unit (compared to conventional toothbrushing). An 18-month clinical study of 20 patients with fixed appliances evaluated elimination of plaque and reduction of gingivitis (Boyd et al 1989). The Rota-Dent proved superior. A direct comparison of both cleaning modes in a crossover investigation is still missing.

One advantage of the Rota-Dent toothbrush over the Interplak device is that the former is much lighter; another relates to the much smaller brush head, which facilitates problem-free access to buccal surfaces of the teeth (Fig 4-23). Access to

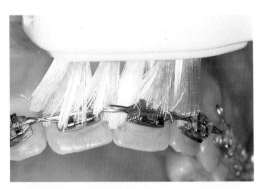

Fig 4-22 The Interplak brush can simplify cleaning of tooth surfaces around brackets and underneath the archwire.

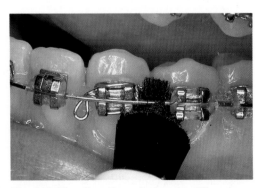

Fig 4-23 The Rota-Dent device simplifies cleaning of teeth for patients with fixed appliances. The brush head is relatively small and the unit is light. However, Rota-Dent use requires greater attention by the patient; simple scrubbing is not sufficient to clean the problematic surfaces.

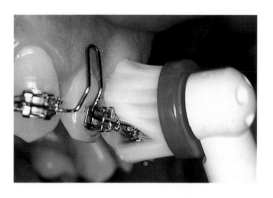

Fig 4-24 It seems difficult to clean under the archwire with a plaque remover device.

these surfaces is significantly more difficult with the Interplak (Levine 1990). On the other hand, the Rota-Dent toothbrush demands greater precision by the patient. Using it for a simple scrubbing technique, as is possible with the Interplak, is entirely useless for efficient cleaning.

For the plaque remover device (Fig 4-24) Braun developed a special brush head for orthodontic patients (OD5). The design of this brush head suggests good cleaning abilities of the tooth surfaces around the attachments. Omitting the second inner bristle tuft circle compared to the regular brush head EB5 obviously allows the outer bristle tufts to reach the tooth surfaces beneath the archwire.

Since no data were available comparing the effectiveness of the above-mentioned electric toothbrushes under at-home conditions, two of the authors (Heintze et al 1996) conducted a single-blind clinical study comprising Interplak, Rota-Dent, and Braun Oral-B Plaque Remover (regular and orthodontic brush head). A manual technique with a conventional toothbrush, an interdental brush, and dental floss (Superfloss) served as reference. Thirty-eight orthodontic patients were randomly allocated to groups that within the test period alternately used the various toothbrushes. Each patient received video and written instructions be-

fore being given a new toothbrush system that was to be used for a period of 4 weeks. For the 4 weeks following, the patients returned to their usual oral hygiene procedures before they were given the next toothbrush.

Oral hygiene was evaluated at the start of each new test period, after 2 weeks and after 4 weeks. Clinical scorings included a modified O'Leary plaque index and Ainamo's gingival bleeding index (Figs 4-25a and 4-25b). Wilcoxon rank test revealed for aggregated surfaces statistically significantly lower plaque scores for Rota-Dent compared to the manual technique (p < 0.001) (Fig 4-26). For all other toothbrushes, no differences were found compared to the manual technique. For plaque indices of specific sites, statistical analysis revealed all electric toothbrushes to be equal to the manual technique.

No differences in gingival bleeding indices were found after 4 weeks with either toothbrush (Fig 4-27). Patients with poor oral hygiene using Rota-Dent and Braun Oral-B Plaque Remover OD5 had statistically significantly lower plaque scores compared to the manual technique (p < 0.01; p < 0.05 respectively); for patients with good oral hygiene, these differences were annulled (Fig 4-28). The brush heads of the various electric brushes showed significant signs of wear after only 4 weeks,

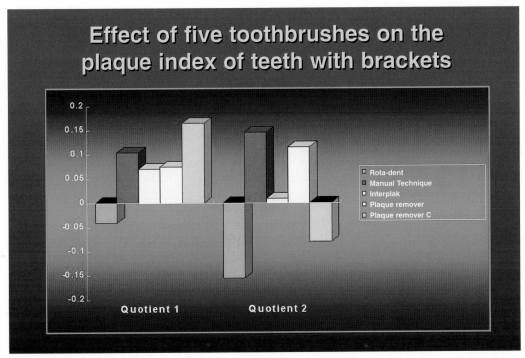

Fig 4-25a Effect of five toothbrushes on the plaque indices of the mesial, buccal, and distal surfaces of teeth with brackets.

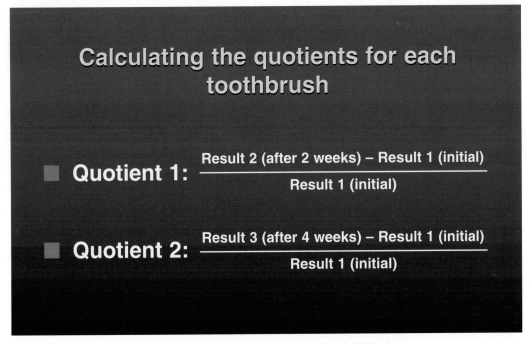

Fig 4-25b Quotients were calculated to account for the varying initial values.

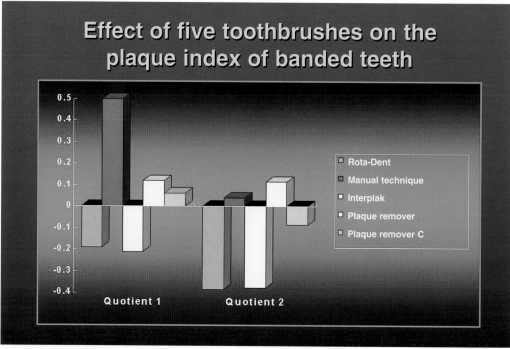

Fig 4-26 Effect of five toothbrushes on the plaque indices of banded teeth.

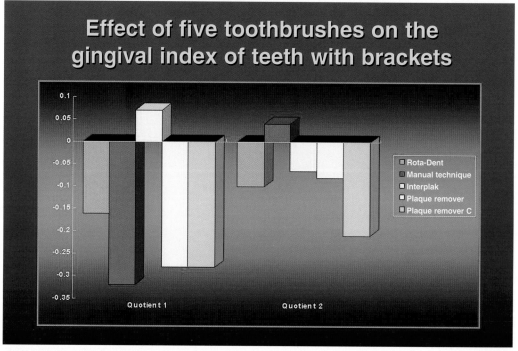

Fig 4-27 Effect of five toothbrushes on the gingival index of the mesial, buccal, and distal tooth surfaces of teeth with brackets.

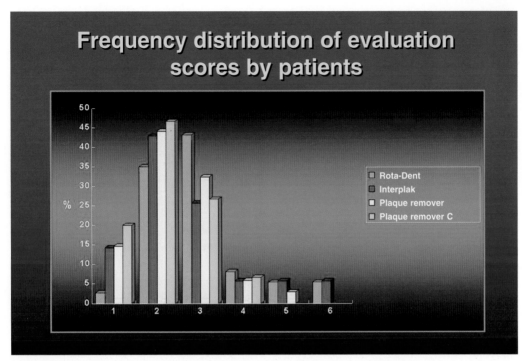

Fig 4-28 Evaluation of four electric toothbrushes: 1 = very good; 6 = very poor.

owing to the speed of brush movement and the retentive elements of fixed appliances (Figs 4-29a and 4-29b).

It can be concluded that:

1. Under at-home conditions, the electric toothbrush Rota-dent without additional devices can contribute to the improvement of oral hygiene in orthodontic patients compared to a manual technique with a hand toothbrush plus interdental brush and dental floss. The same holds true for the Braun Oral-B Plaque Remover with the orthodontic head, but only for patients with poor oral hygiene.

2. Electric toothbrushes can improve patients' motivation, which is very valuable regarding an orthodontic treatment time of 2 years or more. As for personal preference, the majority of the study's participants chose the Braun Oral-B Plaque Remover.

3. Individuals who were highly motivated and well-instructed in a manual technique of oral hygiene (plaque index < 20%) remove their dental plaque regardless of which toothbrush they are given. On the other hand, in patients with poor compliance (PI > 50%) electric devices offer a tool for improving oral hygiene performance.

4. But it must be noted that even after using an electric toothbrush a lot of plaque remains on the teeth surfaces (Fig 4-30).

Figs 4-29a and 4-29b Depending on the frequency of use and the force applied, very different signs of wear appear on the brush heads after 4 weeks' use.

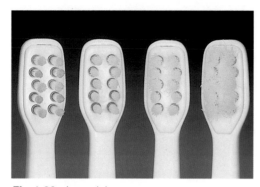

Fig 4-29a Interplak.

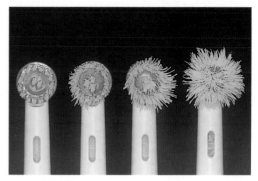

Fig 4-29b Plaque remover device.

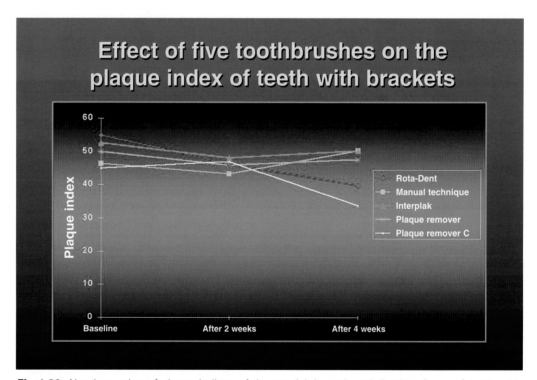

Fig 4-30 Absolute value of plaque indices of the mesial, buccal, and distal surfaces of teeth with bonded brackets as affected by the toothbrushes examined.

MOTIVATION OF THE PATIENT

Before a patient can be motivated to perform oral hygiene, he or she must be told the reason for it. It is important to explain the causes of caries and periodontal disease.

To motivate a patient to perform regular oral hygiene measures, it is necessary to establish a good relationship so that the required information can be passed understandably and clearly. Every dentist and every dental hygienist should take the following rules to heart:

1. In motivating the patient, the dental team should not raise the matter of morals. Usually the patient has a guilty conscience about the matter already, but feelings of guilt rarely motivate.

2. The purpose of the planned program must be explained with precision and in detail.

3. The entire dental team must support the principles of the oral hygiene program.

4. The patient's trust must be won. The patient must have the feeling that he or she understands or can learn everything necessary for prevention, just as thousands of others have done.

5. The patient should become part of a motivational dialogue; the discussion should never be one-sided.

6. Denigrating comments, such as, "I've already explained that to you," must be avoided.

7. A testing atmosphere must be avoided. When the patient demonstrates the brushing technique, corrections should be made without criticism.

8. Every improvement must be verbally rewarded; it is important to build on the positive.

9. All demands made of the patient should be reasonable, so that success is possible. Positive results motivate both sides; failures demotivate.

10. The patient must not gain the impression that something is being forced on him or her. It must be explained that modern prophylaxis is based firmly on recognized research results, and the patient is lucky to learn about them now. The idea is, "We have something to offer to you."

The results of every discussion of prevention should be a silent agreement with the patient, a program to which he or she agrees in recognition of the facts. The following summarizes the manner in which a patient is guided step by step to sensible oral hygiene:

1. The gingival bleeding index (see Fig 2-11) is a good means for motivation. A patient usually associates tissue injury or inflammation with bleeding, which is why he or she pays attention at the site of gingival bleeding. The result should not be overemphasized, however, lest the patient be alarmed. Repeated checking of the gingival bleeding index can be used to demonstrate the patient's success or failure.

2. Disclosure of the plaque is not particularly motivational when used alone. It is a good idea to clean a single tooth, preferably an anterior tooth, professionally. When a disclosing agent is applied, only that tooth is spared its effects.

3. The patient should learn to recognize plaque with his or her tongue. Wherever the tongue feels "furry," plaque remains.

Pharmaceutical Adjuvants for Preventing Caries and Periodontal Disease

5

Pharmaceutical adjuvants are medicaments that support the fundamental therapy. In dentistry, they usually are pastes, liquids, or gels for local application in the oral cavity. These preparations inhibit supragingival plaque formation unspecifically or are directed against specific bacteria in the plaque. The effects of other materials, such as fluorides, are at the saliva-plaque-tooth interface, where they compensate for demineralization. Over the past 20 years, hundreds of publications have discussed the plaque- and gingivitis-reducing effects of antibacterial rinses and dentifrices in vitro and in vivo. Only the topic of fluorides has been discussed as widely.

The selection of the appropriate preparation must be based on the type and severity of the disease. A strict separation between preparations used exclusively for the prevention of gingivitis or periodontitis from those used for the prevention of caries is not possible. Most of the preparations described in this chapter have a plaque-inhibitory effect and therefore are used in prevention of both caries and periodontal disease.

Locally acting pharmaceutical adjuvants must be evaluated for three characteristics:

1. Toxicity should be low. All suitable materials meet this demand. Nevertheless, allergic reactions may occur.
2. The dose-effect profile should be such that very low concentrations at the intended destination are effective.
3. The substantivity should be high; ie, the material should remain in its active form over a long period. Low substantivity often is the reason that a drug with strong activity in vitro fails in vivo.

The seal of the American Dental Association's Council on Dental Therapeutics ("Accepted") can be used as a guideline.

FLUORIDES

Since Dean (1938) initially found a correlation between decreased caries and the natural fluoride content of drinking water, numerous forms of fluoride have been proposed for caries prevention. Dental textbooks have tended to classify these into two categories:

1. Fluoride ingested orally and absorbed in the stomach.
2. Fluorides applied locally or topically to the teeth.

The first group includes fluoride supplements; the second includes toothpastes containing fluorides, oral rinses, gels, and dental materials that release fluoride over a long period (eg, denture resins, glass-ionomer cements, composite sealants, restorative materials, and adhesives for orthodontic attachments).

This type of classification into systemic and local action is inappropriate today, because overlaps occur. As soon as the first teeth erupt, the (fluoridated) water in which rice has been cooked, for example, also has a local effect on the teeth; locally applied fluorides, eg, in dentifrices or oral rinses, are swallowed, particularly by children, and thus act systemically, too.

Fundamentally, it may be postulated that the more frequently fluorides are used, the better. In all cases, however, the single dose must be determined in accordance with dose frequency. If fluorides are used daily, high dosage is not necessary and may even be harmful.

Fluoride supplements

Fluoride supplements are substances to which fluoride, usually in the form of sodium fluoride, has been added. Water, table salt, milk, sugar, juices, tablets, drops, and chewing gum are among the carriers suitable for fluoride. The most examined and controlled form of fluoride supplementation is fluoridated drinking water. Depending on the climate zone, optimal concentration is between 0.7 and 1.2 ppm. In hot regions, the fluoride concentration must be reduced because of the greater intake of liquids; in cooler climates, it must be increased because fluid intake is lower. The fluoride concentration often is adjusted to seasonal temperature variations.

About 300 million individuals around the world use fluoridated drinking water today; to this group are added the approximately 103 million people whose drinking water is naturally fluoridated at about 0.7 ppm (WHO 1986). In the United States alone, 135 million people (55% of the population) use drinking water systems containing fluoride. Forty-two of the 50 largest cities in the United States have fluoridated drinking water. According to a report of the Fédération Dentaire Internationale (FDI/WHO 1985), 39 nations around the world provide some fluoridation of drinking water.

The caries-reducing effect of fluoridated drinking water has been confirmed in countless studies. Caries reduction is about 40% in the primary and 50% to 60% in the permanent dentition (review Murray 1993). Caries prevalence has been reduced in children and adolescents in most industrialized nations over the past 20 to 25 years. This decrease was independent of water fluoridation (Murray 1993). As the use of preparations containing fluoride (toothpastes, fluoride tablets, fluoride rinses, fluoridated salt, fluoride gels and varnishes, etc) increased, the differences in caries prevalence between communities with or without fluoridated drinking water became smaller (O'Mullane 1990).

More recent studies from the United States, Ireland, New Zealand, and Brazil show caries reduction of only 29% to 35% attributable to water fluoridation (Newbrun 1989; Heintze et al 1997). This limited caries reduction also may be explained by the fact that inhabitants of communities without fluoridated water ingest fluoridated foods and liquids produced in communities with fluoridated water (Hattab and Wei 1988).

Fluoridation of drinking water is being criticized increasingly today. It is not held to be generally needed, because caries rates in children and adolescents have been reduced; fluoride is even considered harmful because of the increase in dental fluorosis. The seriousness of dental fluorosis is related closely to the fluoride content of drinking water; many studies have demonstrated a linear relationship (eg, Fejerskov et al 1990). A series of publications, however, have proven high prevalence of fluorosis even in regions with low (0.2 ppm) fluoride concentrations in drinking water. This observation is explained by the fact that individuals in such regions are exposed to additional sources of fluoride.

The minor increase in fluorosis in Western Europe, the United States, Australia, and New Zealand (Pendrys and Stamm 1990) is ascribed to the effects of locally or systemically acting fluorides, or both. Over recent decades, such materials have been used with increasing frequency, particularly in the form of toothpastes and tablets. Significant systemic effects of fluoridated toothpaste must be assumed in children younger than 6 years old, because they swallow much of the dentifrice (Dowell 1981). Because locally applied fluoride is effective in even very low concentrations, some authors have suggested that the fluoride concentration in children's toothpaste be reduced to less than 300 ppm. That proposal has been implemented in some European nations.

Nevertheless, administration of fluoride tablets is indicated until the 13th year of life, if the fluoride concentration in drinking water is less than 0.3 ppm. Only in this way is sufficient fluoride made available to promote remineralization of primary and permanent teeth equally. The decisive factor is not the preeruptive effect of fluoride from intestinal resorption, but rather the posteruptive local effect directly on the dental enamel. To achieve maximum effect, the patient should slowly chew or suck the tablets. Fluoride drops are available for infants (0.125 mg F^-/tablet).

Fluoride tablets commonly are prescribed for children from the first to the 13th year of life. Split-dose administration should be prescribed to provide 0.25 mg fluoride per administration. Not only are peak plasma levels reduced in this way, but the fluoride is deposited locally more frequently. The administration of fluoride is more important than splitting the dose, however (Widenheim 1982). If drinking water is optimally fluoridated (0.7 to 1.2 ppm, depending on average climate temperature), supplemental fluoride administration should not be recommended. If the fluoride concentration of drinking water is less than 0.7 ppm, fluoride tablets should be prescribed in accordance with the child's age, weight, and fluoride concentration in the water, according to Newbrun (1992), as indicated in Table 5-1.

Table 5-1 Flouride tablet administration based on fluoride in drinking water

Age (y)	Weight (kg)	< 0.3 ppm F^-(mg)	0.3 – 0.7 ppm F^-(mg)	> 0.7 ppm F^-(mg)
0–2	3.4–12.4	0.25	0.00	0.00
2–4	12.4–16.4	0.50	0.25	0.00
4–6	16.4–21.5	0.75	0.50	0.00
6–13	> 21.5	1.00	0.75	0.00

From Newbrun 1992.

Despite these guidelines, studies in the United States indicate that nearly 80% of all children up to age 6 have been given fluoride tablets, even in regions with optimally fluoridated water supplies (Pendrys and Morse 1990). Such inappropriate prescribing is surely responsible, at least in part, for the recent increase in fluorosis (Clark 1994). A "window of vulnerability" (Newbrun 1992) for fluorosis of the permanent anterior teeth is open between birth and the 6th year of life. In prescribing fluoride tablets, the dentist should probably orient the dose more to the child's weight than to his or her age. The threshold value for formation of fluorosis is approximately 0.05 mg F^-/kg body weight (Burt 1992).

Fluoridation of table salt is a true alternative to fluoridation of drinking water. That is particularly true for nations in which fluoridation of the drinking water is expensive, difficult to carry out, or illegal. Fluoridated table salt containing 250 mg F^-/kg is available in certain European and Latin American nations. It is important that the consumer can be able to choose between fluoridated and nonfluoridated salt, so that the "forced medication" argument, sometimes raised against fluoridation of drinking water, is avoided. At 50%, the caries reduction afforded by fluoridated salt is similar to that of fluoridated water (Marthaler et al 1978).

Because milk is a valuable basic food, particularly for infants and children, fluoridation of milk provided in schools was proposed in the 1950s. Calcium and proteins, however, seem to reduce the local availability of fluoride in milk, lowering the likely caries-reducing effect below that of drinking water or salt (Duff 1981). Few studies have been published about fluoridated milk. The World Health Organization sees an underutilized potential and supports products in Great Britain, eastern Europe, Latin America, and China (WHO/BDMF 1993).

Fluoride rinses

As soon as children have learned to rinse, the change from fluoride tablets to rinses containing fluoride may be considered. The 6th year of life should be regarded the lower age limit. Rinses ordinarily contain 0.025% to 0.050% sodium fluoride, 0.025% amine fluoride, 0.010% zinc fluoride, or 0.020% acidulated phosphate fluoride (APF). Caries reduction with fluoride rinses in general is in the order of 30%, if 10 mL of rinse is swished in the mouth for at least 1 minute daily (Newbrun 1992).

To manage the problem of cooperation, oral rinse programs were introduced into Swedish schools as early as the 1970s. Usually, rinsing was practiced under supervision at weekly or biweekly sessions. The need for such programs may be questioned today in light of decreasing caries rates and the availability of other fluoride sources. Some Scandinavian nations already have halted such programs entirely, because examinations of patients with low caries activity revealed no added effect (Poulsen et al 1984, Axelsson et al 1987).

This finding does not apply, however, to patients with fixed orthodontic appliances. Relevant studies have shown that daily use of a fluoride rinse during the active treatment phase does, indeed, reduce the incidence of initial caries lesions. A study found initial carious lesions of various sizes in only 7.5% of 1567 teeth; furthermore, only one cavitation was found (Geiger et al 1988). Comparison with a control group showed this to be an improvement of 25%, even though patient cooperation was poor. How much better might the results have been if patient co-operation had been good? More highly concentrated solutions are recommended for patients with increased caries risk (Zachrisson 1975).

In the 1980s, a rinse containing amine fluoride plus zinc fluoride (Meridol) was developed. Its use reportedly led to significantly better plaque reduction than did a placebo preparation (Brecx et al 1990). This preparation appears to be particularly advantageous because zinc fluoride has a stronger inhibitory effect on *Streptococcus mutans* than does sodium fluoride. A comparative study by Klock et al (1985) indicated that twice daily rinsing with a zinc fluoride solution led to low *S mutans* rates even after 2 years; the frequency of caries and gingivitis was also lower in the zinc fluoride group than in the control group treated with sodium fluoride. Nevertheless, the caries-inhibitory effect of zinc fluoride solutions has been questioned (Mellberg 1990).

The other component of Meridol is amine fluoride, which, as an organic fluoride, has a stronger caries-protective effect than inorganic fluoride. A clinical study by Renggli (1983) indicated that a rinse containing amine fluoride and zinc fluoride, with a fluoride concentration of 100 ppm, inhibited plaque formation approximately as well as a 0.2% solution of chlorhexidine.

Meridol may lead to tooth discoloration, which is ascribed to the zinc fluoride (Fig 5-1). The discolorations are limited exclusively to the outer layer of the enamel and correlate with oral hygiene. The worse the patient's oral hygiene, the more likely there is to be tooth discoloration. These discolorations are not, however, as intensive as those resulting from chlorhexidine and occur in only about 10% of patients.

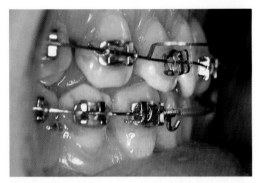

Fig 5-1 Regular use of Meridol can lead to reversible discoloration of the superficial enamel layer after a short time.

Fluoride gels

Gels containing fluoride are placed on patients annually or semiannually in the dental office. Some authors also promote the idea of brushing weekly with the gels. Such gels contain fluoride in high concentration: 2.00% sodium fluoride, 8.00% zinc fluoride, APF with 1.23% fluoride, or 1.25% fluoride as a combination of amine fluoride and zinc fluoride. Acidulated phosphate fluoride, treated with phosphoric acid, increases the uptake of fluoride into the enamel because of its low pH. Used especially in the United States and certain European nations, APF is applied for 4 minutes in a disposable tray. Previous cleaning is not required, because fluoride uptake by the enamel is not disturbed by plaque or tooth epithelium (Ripa et al 1983). Because APF attacks the glass components of restorations, it should not be used repeatedly in patients with glass-containing restorations. The average caries reduction provided by fluoride gels is approximately 30% (Marthaler 1988). Gels containing amine fluoride are used almost exclusively in Europe, both professionally by the dentist and by the patient at home. The caries reduction afforded by such gels is of the same order as that of other fluoride compounds (Ripa 1990).

Excessive application of fluoride in high concentrations, as is found in gels, may cause fluorosis or fluoride intoxication. Two plastic trays for simultaneous placement on the maxilla and the mandible, a practice that should be followed only in the dental office, contain approximately 20 mL of gel, corresponding to 250 mg fluoride if the fluoride concentration is 1.25%.

At least until the 6th year of life, fluoride should not be used at such a high concentration (Horowitz 1977). Studies have shown that gel preparations with lower fluoride concentrations are equally effective (Sluiter and Purdell-Lewis 1984). These also prevent the patient from swallowing of large amounts of fluoride, which is a significant risk with all preparations that have higher fluoride concentrations (Ekstrand and Koch 1980). Only custom trays with a sealing rim should be used.

While the trays are in the mouth, suction should be applied continuously. Immediately thereafter, the patient should be told to rinse for one minute. Effective rinsing can reduce the amount of intraorally retained fluoride to 8% (LeCompte and Doyle 1982). The home use of fluoride gels, whether in trays or by brushing, should be avoided, at least during childhood. Independently of the toxicologic considerations, all preparations with high fluoride concentration share another disadvantage: They cause excessive fluoride enrichment of the outer enamel layers and thus lead to only superficial closure of the demineralized zones. In practice, this prevents profound penetration of fluoride and deep remineralization (Silverstone et al 1981, ten Cate et al 1981, Arends and Christoffersen 1990). Surface remineralization may be sufficient for primary protection against caries, but treatment of initial lesions (white-spot lesions) with high fluoride concentration materials today is poor dental practice.

The permanent presence of fluorides is important, especially in patients who have fixed orthodontic appliances. Microhardness tests on enamel have shown significantly higher values in patients who have received fluoride applications regularly. The results were compared to those in control patients who did not receive supplemental fluorides (O'Reilly and Featherstone 1987). The enamel of the control group had an average demineralization of 15% at a depth of 50 μm; whereas the enamel was defect less due to continuous remineralization in the test group; irrespective whether fluoride rinses or gels were used.

Fluoride varnishes

Fluoride varnishes were developed to increase the contact time between fluoride and enamel and thus to promote the formation of fluorapatite. They also act like other fluoride preparations, through slow release of loosely bound fluoride (Øgaard et al 1984). They provide caries reduction of 30%, similar to that achieved through other methods of fluoride administration (De Bruyn and Arends 1987). The great advantage of such varnishes lies in the fact that they are effective when applied two to four times per year. Thus their cost-benefit ratio is better than that of gels. Varnishes also eliminate the potential problem of poor compliance, because they are applied professionally.

Two products are available at present: Duraphat and Fluor Protector. Duraphat contains 2.26% fluoride in an alcoholic solution of natural resins. The product is water tolerant and therefore also coats moist teeth with a well-adhering film. This property increases the period of activity by a matter of hours. Even diffusion in sound enamel is possible to some extent (Seppä et al 1982). Fluoride ions are released slowly into the oral cavity. Only small bits of resin that do not produce peak fluoride loads are swallowed (Ekstrand et al 1980). Nonetheless, Duraphat is a highly concentrated fluoride material; just 1 mL contains approximately 23 mg of fluoride, which corresponds to 110 0.25 mg fluoride tablets.

Duraphat is used predominantly in Europe and Canada, particularly by public health services. More recently it has been permitted in the United States. Weekly oral rinse programs have been replaced by semiannual Duraphat applications in some Scandinavian nations after higher caries reduction rates were reported (Koch et al 1979, Seppä and Pöllänen 1987). Another study, however, found no difference between Duraphat and oral rinses (Kirkegaard et al 1986).

Fluor Protector, a fluoride varnish of a different type, was developed by Arends and Schuthof (1975). In a polyurethane base, it contains 0.1% fluoride in the form of difluorosilane. The liquid, provided in ampules or screw top bottles containing 1 or 0.4 mL respectively, is applied as shown in Figs 5-2a to 5-2c.

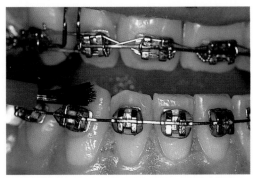

Fig 5-2a Fluor Protector is applied to the teeth with a brush after prophylaxis is completed and adequate isolation is achieved.

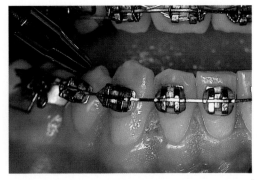

Fig 5-2b Fluor Protector is dispersed over the surface with an air stream.

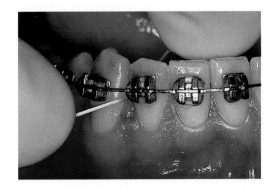

Fig 5-2c Dental floss has proven the best means for dispersing the material evenly in the proximal spaces.

Fluor Protector is self-curing and clear when polymerized. The fluorosilane in Fluor Protector is insoluble in water but reacts when in contact with saliva. It forms a dense, thick calcium fluoride layer that becomes water soluble after sugar impulses and the resulting acid formation by bacteria. Over a period of 2 to 3 months, it releases very small amounts of hydrogen fluoride, which penetrates easily and deeply into the enamel (Arends and Schuthof 1975).

In an in vivo study (De Bruyn and Buskes 1988), in which patients wore experimental "window dentures" fitted with enamel slices previously impregnated for 24 hours with Fluor Protector or Duraphat, microradiographic analyses showed the mineral loss of enamel treated with Fluor Protector to be much less than that of the Duraphat-treated specimens. This result has been ascribed to the significantly greater amount of fluoride deposited on the enamel by Fluor Protector, among other things (De Bruyn and Arends 1987).

Long-term clinical studies of the caries-protective effect of these varnishes, in contrast, indicate Duraphat to be somewhat more effective than Fluor Protector (Clark et al 1985, Seppä and Pöllänen 1987). Nevertheless, results of a 3-year study by Axelsson et al (1987) indicate that use of Fluor Protector at 3-months intervals led to significantly greater reduction in proximal caries than did weekly supervised rinsing with an 0.5% solution of sodium fluoride. However, fluoride rinses were provided at weekly intervals, and professional prophylaxis was provided before each application of Fluor Protector. Thus, the at-risk surfaces were freed of plaque; such intensive cleaning is not routinely provided.

Adriaens et al (1990) were able to demonstrate the caries-inhibiting effect of Fluor Protector in a clinical study with 28 patients with fixed appliances. The molars on one side of the arch, treated with Fluor Protector before band placement, had fewer initial caries lesions than did those in the untreated side. The teeth had been isolated carefully before application of Fluor Protector and band placement.

Although Fluor Protector shows good results in vitro, good clinical results are not always achieved; desired clinical effects are produced only when the prerequisites for use (clean, dry teeth) are provided. The Dry Field System, a combination lip, cheek, and tongue retractor with an integrated saliva ejector (Jost-Brinkmann and Miethke 1988), can be useful in providing sufficient field dryness. The prerequisites for successful application of Fluor Protector can be met by drying the surfaces of all teeth and consequently placing the solution with a brush.

It is not desirable to coat all accessible tooth surfaces with a fluoride varnish. Rather, applications should be limited to surfaces at risk, including occlusal surfaces, particularly those in the eruption stage; proximal surfaces, especially of posterior teeth; exposed root surfaces; surfaces around brackets; and margins of restorations/bands. Fluoride varnishes also are useful on sensitive tooth cervices.

Duraphat acts as a sealant on occlusal surfaces in the eruption stage. For example, in a study by Holm et al (1984), a single application of Duraphat to erupting first molars led to a 56% reduction in fissure caries. Application of Duraphat in carpules is desirable, because the syringe tip can be placed under the remaining integument (Figs 5-3a and 5-3b). Whether distribution of the material with dental floss provides additional protection remains unclear.

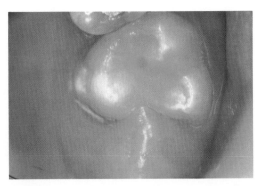

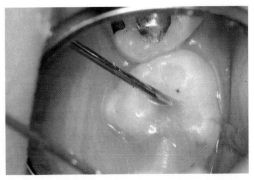

Fig 5-3a During eruption of the maxillary first molar, the fissures are particularly at risk for caries because of increased plaque retention and poor accessibility.

Fig 5-3b A fluoride varnish is applied under the integument of an erupting first molar.

Professional prophylaxis before application of fluoride varnish is not required unconditionally, because the fluoride ions permeate a thin layer of plaque without difficulty (Ripa et al 1983). Although Duraphat may be applied even to moist tooth surfaces to form a hard film, it is better to dry the teeth beforehand. This not only simplifies application, but also appears to improve fluoride uptake by the enamel (Koch et al 1988). When Fluor Protector is used, drying of the tooth surfaces is crucial to the caries-protective effect.

The patient must not eat or drink anything or brush the teeth for 2 to 4 hours after the varnish is applied, so that it can interact with the enamel. No scientific verification of this recommendation has been reported.

As the kinetics of fluoride effects have become better understood, the frequency of topical fluoride application has been adjusted. Some time ago, it was believed that such treatments were required three to six times annually because the loosely bound fluoride would be washed away. At present, it appears that two applications per year suffice (Seppä and Tolonen 1989). More frequent application appears in order for patients with fixed appliances because of the increased threat of caries posed by the numerous retention elements.

Fluoride-releasing adhesives

Effective caries prophylaxis with fluorides is achieved through the continuous presence of low concentrations of fluoride ions. In recognition of this fact, various dental materials that release fluoride over longer periods have been developed in the recent past. In addition to the glass-ionomer cements used for cementing bands and brackets, various bracket adhesives (eg, Fluorobond, Excel, and Light Bond) release fluoride ions. Numerous studies have demonstrated that initial lesions and caries are effectively reduced when such resin composites are used (Sonis and Snell 1989, Underwood et al 1989, Hiller et al 1990).

How do such materials rank in durability and mechanical strength? A study by Underwood et al (1989) indicated that clinical failures are as frequent as are found with ordinary resin composites, the fracture sites being, as usual, at the enamel-composite interface. In a study by McCourt et al (1991), the adhesive force of another fluoride-releasing bracket adhesive was less than a third the adhesive bond strength of ordinary adhesives after 30 days in place. These contradictory results are presumably mainly due to the different materials tested.

To prevent the initial lesions that often are found following removal of brackets, treatment with highly concentrated acidic fluorides (eg, amine fluorides) before bracket placement has been suggested (Wang and Sheen 1991). According to these authors, the adhesive strength of brackets following this procedure is similar to that found in teeth with untreated enamel. Even application of 2% to 4% sodium fluoride solution after etching, immediately before bonding, has no significant effect on the tensile and the shear bond strengths of the adhesive material (Bishara et al 1989). Indeed, etching increases fluoride uptake in dental enamel (Valk et al 1985).

A polymethyl methacrylate resin (Orthocryl Plus) was developed for removable devices for the same reason. It releases calcium fluoride in low concentration over a long period (Miethke and Newesely 1988).

CHLORHEXIDINE

Chlorhexidine, a strongly alkaline diguanidine derivative, is one of the safest and most effective antiseptics known. It is a nonspecific antimicrobial agent that does not disturb the healing process even when placed on an open wound.

Mechanisms of action and properties

Briefly stated, the mechanisms of action of chlorhexidine are as follows:

1. It impedes adhesion of bacteria on the tooth surface.
2. It is absorbed by the cell wall of bacteria, inhibiting bacterial proliferation.
3. It is as effective against gram-negative bacteria as it is against mutans streptococci but less against lactobacilli.
4. It has great substantivity; the positively charged molecule is bound not only to tooth surfaces but also to mucosa, and the active form is released over a long period.

Because chlorhexidine is released slowly, it hinders adhesion of bacteria to the tooth surface (Lang 1978). Rinsing twice daily with an 0.2% chlorhexidine solution reduces the total bacterial count in saliva by 85% to 90% (Löe et al 1972). According to their study, if chlorhexidine is used over a brief period, the plaque indices drop dramatically; the effect on existing gingivitis is less strongly apparent. The best results for treatment of gingivitis are obtained when chlorhexidine is used in conjunction with controlled oral hygiene.

Chlorhexidine is very efficient as a cariostatic material because it acts not only against gram-negative bacteria, but also against yeasts and gram-positive bacteria, such as *Streptococcus mutans* and *Streptococcus sobrinus* (Emilson 1981). Therefore it is not surprising that the effect of chlorhexidine, in terms of reduced caries incidence, was clearly higher than that of fluorides in comparative clinical studies (Lindquist et al 1988). The inhibitory effect of chlorhexidine on *S mutans* also was confirmed in patients with fixed orthodontic appliances (Lundström and Krasse 1987).

It is appropriate to ask, despite the obviously positive effects of chlorhexidine, whether such a reduction of the oral flora leads to a massive negative effect on the ecological balance. Does it lead, perhaps, to overgrowth of other, resistant organisms or, given long use, to resistance of those organisms that were originally intended to be eliminated? In fact, a study has shown that the effect on existing gingivitis is only temporary (Curtress et al 1977). Presumably, organisms that became resistant can proliferate again over time and induce gingivitis.

Unpleasant side effects, such as discoloration of teeth and resin composite restorations as well as bracket adhesives (Fig 5-4) and increased calculus formation, occur with long-term use. Elastics and orthodontic chains, however, do not stain when using chlorhexidine (Fadel et al 1992). The extent of the discoloration can be reduced by intensive toothbrushing; discoloration is less extensive in children than in adults (Lang 1978). Another disadvantage of chlorhexidine, independent of the duration of use, is its unpleasant taste. The bitter taste can be masked by the addition of flavoring agents, which, however, reduce the effectiveness of chlorhexidine by 30% to 40% (Lang 1978).

Attempts have been made to overcome the problems of discoloration and taste through use of other dosage forms. A chewing gum containing sorbitol and 0.375% to 0.625% chlorhexidine acetate, chewed twice daily for 10 minutes reduces plaque proliferation as effectively as rinsing with chlorhexidine solution two times a day (Ainamo et al 1990). Lozenges with 5 mg chlorhexidine dihydrochloride, used three times daily after toothbrushing, can prohibit plaque accumulation up to 76%

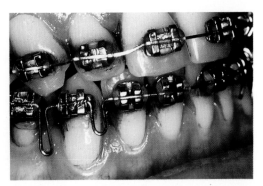

Fig 5-4 Chlorhexidine can cause reversible tooth discoloration with long use.

without tooth discoloration or disturbances of taste (Kaufman et al 1989).

The possibility of systemic side effects of long-term treatment has also been examined. Schiött et al (1976) found no deviations in blood and urine values from normal patients in probands who used chlorhexidine permanently for 2 years. As is true for all medicaments, long-term safety depends on dosage: 0.1% to 0.2% solutions are sufficient, and these concentrations should not be exceeded (Lang et al 1982).

Oral rinse

The oral rinse is a dosage form used especially frequently in dentistry, for patients with gingivitis and periodontitis as well as before and after surgical procedures, for example. Ready-to-use 0.1% or 0.2% solutions (eg, Peridex) are available. To achieve the desired effect, rinsing should last for at least 20 to 45 seconds. This ensures that at least 30% of the chlorhexidine is bound to the oral mucosa (Bonesvoll et al 1974). Professionals may inject oral rinse solutions directly into inflamed pockets.

Chlorhexidine solution in an oral irrigator can be particularly useful for patients with fixed orthodontic appliances (Lang and Räber 1981) and is better, in any case, than simple rinsing. In a 6-month study, the combination of an 0.06% solution (Peridex) and the Water-Pik was more effective in prevention of gingivitis than was rinsing with an 0.12% solution or "normal" oral hygiene or the Water-Pik with water only (Flemming et al 1990). Intraoral spray devices distribute pharmaceutical adjuvants so well that the active ingredients can even permeate gingival pockets (Eakle et al 1986).

Gel

If only the cariogenic effect of chlorhexidine is required, treatment with a gel is more effective than treatment with an oral rinse, because the gel adheres to the tooth surface for a longer period. The gel (eg, Corsodyl gel, 1% chlorhexidine) can be applied with a toothbrush or in a custom-made tray (Figs 5-5a to 5-5e). Use of the custom tray provides even distribution of the gel, and the material reaches the surfaces of the teeth without dilution; it is not distributed over the mucosal surfaces, as is the case for oral rinse solutions. The gel leads to significant reduction in mutans streptococci, while the patient's sense of taste is impaired only slightly.

To reduce the *S mutans* count drastically, Krasse (1986) proposed use of custom trays filled with 1% chlorhexidine gel to a depth sufficient to cover all tooth surfaces. This dosage form reduces *S mutans* more than does distribution of an equal amount of gel with a toothbrush over the period of 1 week (Ostela et al 1990).

Certain problems of gel therapy must be overcome in patients with fixed orthodontic appliances. For example, the custom trays must be fabricated by blocking out the regions of the attachments on the cast (see Fig 5-5a) or even before the intraoral impression is made (see Fig 5-5b). A material that remains soft (eg, Erkoflex or Bioplast 2.0 mm) is desirable for use as the tray.

After placement of the tray filled with gel, the patient should chew on the tray for 5 minutes so that the gel is distributed in the interdental spaces and around the brackets. Spread of the material is enhanced by the use of tray material that remains soft; it has the effect of a pump. Direct contact of the gel with the teeth is a critical factor, however, because the gel diffuses less than the oral rinse (Saxén et al 1976). It is best for the patient to apply the chlorhexidine just before bedtime, so that the material can exert its full effect for the entire night.

To achieve optimum effect, this intensive chlorhexidine therapy should be provided daily for 2 weeks. Two centimeters of 1% gel corresponds to 10 mL of 0.2% solution; thus, 20 mg of chlorhexidine are available in both dosage forms (Lang and Brecx 1986).

If the required cooperation of the patient and his or her parents over the 2-week period cannot be assured, a more drastic version of this treatment is possible. The patient chews in the doctors operatory on filled trays three times for 5 minutes on 2 consecutive days, rinsing thoroughly with water between chewing periods.

The tray therapy is inappropriate for very young children, because they resist introduction of the trays into the mouth, perceiving the trays as foreign bodies, and because they are likely to swallow much of the gel. For such patients, the gel should be applied with a toothbrush or a cotton roll.

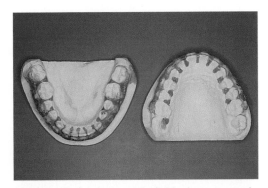

Fig 5-5a To fabricate an individual tray to apply chlorhexidine gel in a patient with fixed appliances, the brackets, bands, and archwires must be blocked out with wax on the casts.

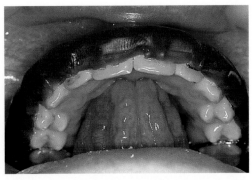

Fig 5-5b Alternatively, the attachments may be covered in the mouth, which facilitates the taking of an alginate impression.

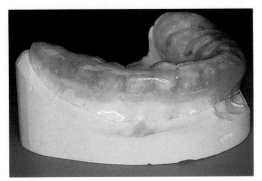

Fig 5-5c The completed tray for the mandible. If a wax that melts at high temperatures is used, the splint can be formed directly over the wax.

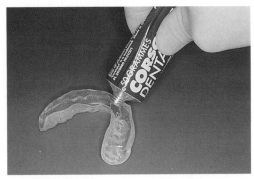

Fig 5-5d Chlorhexidine gel is applied sparingly to the custom tray.

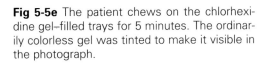

Fig 5-5e The patient chews on the chlorhexidine gel–filled trays for 5 minutes. The ordinarily colorless gel was tinted to make it visible in the photograph.

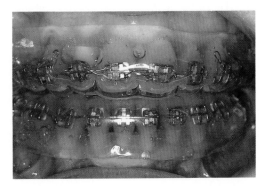

After effective chlorhexidine treatment, the mutans streptococci values decrease rapidly and remain at low levels for 2 to 4 months (Emilson 1981, Ostela et al 1990). Thus, the clinician gains sufficient time to eliminate the ecological niches for the organism during the stages of motivation and instruction in oral hygiene, diet counseling, and some form of fluoride therapy. During this period, of course, necessary restorative measures should be completed.

The success of chlorhexidine was made clear by a study by Zickert et al (1982). Forty-eight children whose salivary mutans streptococci values were higher than 250,000 colony forming units per milliliter of saliva were selected from a group of 101 13- to 14-year-old children and treated with 1% chlorhexidine gel daily for 2 weeks. Three years later, the test group averaged 3.9 new carious lesions, while the untreated controls (ie, those given no specific antimicrobial therapy) had an average of 20.8 new lesions.

A recently published meta-analysis (summary of different clinical studies by means of a clearly structured and defined statistical approach) determined the caries-inhibiting effect of chlorhexidine to be 46% (van Rijkom et al 1996). The more drastic chlorhexidine therapy described must be provided in its entirety (six applications over 2 days). The Ostela et al (1990) study showed that, after a single application of chlorhexidine, mutans streptococci could not adhere to the Dentocult SM strip, but they could be cultivated on mitis-salivarius agar. Thus, a negative strip test result with the Dentocult SM strip after a single application of chlorhexidine gel should not be interpreted as a sign to discontinue the medication. To determine the actual effect of chlorhexidine, the Dentocult SM strip test should be made 2 weeks after the end of chlorhexidine treatment at the earliest. Only then do remaining mutans streptococci rods attach to the test strips, so that the test provides dependable information of the actual bacterial count.

The number of S mutans colonies should be checked at regular intervals. That is especially important during orthodontic treatment, because this group of bacteria recolonizes quickly in the numerous niches present in the form of bands and brackets (Lundström and Krasse 1987) (Fig 5-6).

The action of chlorhexidine gel is increased when combined with a fluoride gel, as was shown in an in vitro study. The combination with amine fluoride is superior to that with sodium fluoride (Ostela and Tenovuo 1990). A high-dose combination of amine fluoride and zinc fluoride (1.2% fluoride total) without chlorhexidine, however, was most inhibitory against S mutans and S sobrinus in that study. Only chlorhexidine, it should be noted, was also effective against lactobacilli. These in vitro results have not been confirmed in vivo.

Varnish

Over the last 10 years varnishes have been developed that contain chlorhexidine. Three are commercially available: EC40 (Explore) with 40% chlorhexidine, Chlorzoin (Knowell) with 10% chlorhexidine, and Cervitec (Vivadent) containing 1% chlorhexidine and 1% thymol. Thymol also has an antimicrobial effect and is specifically directed toward those organisms not impaired by chlorhexidine (Huizinga et al 1991). The solvent of Cervitec evaporates within 5 minutes after application, and the amount of chlorhexidine and thymol increases to almost 8%.

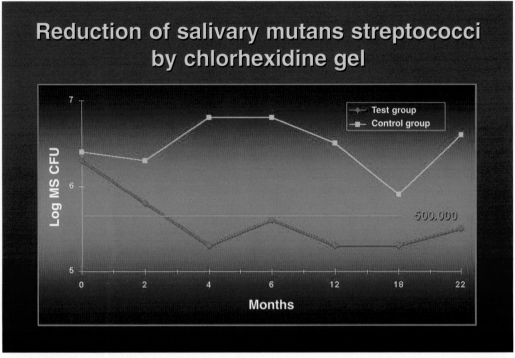

Fig 5-6 Effect of chlorhexidine gel treatment on the mutans streptococci count in the saliva of treated and untreated patients. (Redrawn from Lundström and Krasse 1987.)

With confocal laser scanning microscopy, it was found that Cervitec penetrates 50% (maximum) into tubules of demineralized dentin (Arends et al 1997). In vitro studies under extreme cariogenic conditions showed that after a single application of Cervitec, caries was reduced by up to 43% in enamel and up to 80% in cementum in comparison to a control group (Huizinga 1991).

Chlorhexidine varnishes are only applied on surfaces at risk (eg, those around brackets, proximal and root surfaces). These varnishes have the advantage of releasing chlorhexidine over a prolonged period of time. Therefore, treatment can be repeated within extended intervals. For Cervitec, at least three applications within 3 weeks seem to be more effective in suppressing mutans streptococci than three monthly applications (Twetman and Petersson 1997). In patients with fixed appliances, 1 week after the first varnish application mutans streptococci were found in only 33% of the plaque samples compared to 78% of those treated with a placebo (Twetman et al 1995). After the second application (1 month later) the figures were 53% and 88%, respectively.

The frequency of applications is crucial for long-term suppression of bacteria. At least a bimonthly application routine (three times each) is needed in patients with fixed appliances, whereas in patients with removable appliances a 3-month routine seems to be sufficient (Petersson et al 1991). However, suppression of bacteria prior to bracket bonding might be more promising. When Chlorzoin was applied four times before insertion of the appliance, mutans streptococci were not detected in 11 out of 26 patients even after 7-months (Sandham et al 1992). Therefore, when administering Chlorzoin in high-risk patients, four weekly initial applications are recommended. As far as EC40 is concerned, a single application of the varnish may be sufficient in maintaining the level of mutans streptococci for at least 3 months (Schaeken et al 1991). Due to its lower content of chlorhexidine, recolonization of mutans streptococci is more rapid with Cervitec than with EC40, thus requiring more frequent applications (Petersson et al 1991).

For all treatments involving antibacterial varnishes, microbial growth should be monitored site-specifically (eg with Dentocult SM strip), since plaque reduction around the brackets or proximal surfaces is not adequately reflected in whole saliva samples (Twetman et al 1997).

Before any varnish is applied, dental plaque should be removed and the teeth isolated with cotton rolls and dried with air. The varnish is either applied with a brush or, more conveniently, with a disposable pipette (Cervitec, Chlorzoin) or by means of carpules and a syringe (EC40). Subsequently, Cervitec and Chlorzoin are dispersed over the surfaces and dried with a stream of air (Fig 5-7). Cervitec and EC40 set as soon as the varnish comes into contact with saliva. The Cervitec coat will be colorless, in contrast to EC40, which will create a chewing-gum-like white film that has to be removed after 10 minutes with curettes and/or rotating brushes. Chlorzoin, however, must be covered with an adhesive (polyurethane).

Since EC40 has a high concentration of chlorhexidine, contact with mucosal tissues should be avoided so as not to cause

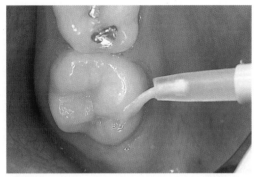

Fig 5-7 After relative isolation is achieved, Cervitec, a chlorhexidine varnish, is distributed over the surface of the tooth and dried with a stream of air.

irritations. However, such irritations seldom occur. More often patients complain of a bad taste and burning sensation.

No staining of teeth or composite resin has been observed for any of the varnishes if prophylaxis is performed prior to the application. If not, a slight brown staining may appear, especially when using Chlorzoin. After Cervitec or Chlorzoin is applied, the patient should refrain from eating for 4 hours, from toothbrushing for 24 hours, and from flossing for 3 days. The varnish invariably will come off the teeth over the next few days after treatment.

The question of whether application of a chlorhexidine varnish is superior to a chlorhexidine gel treatment remains unanswered. One study indicates that a chlorhexidine-containing toothpaste (Parosan, 0.4% chlorhexidine), a gel with 1% chlorhexidine (Corsodyl), and Cervitec were equally effective in reducing mutans streptococci in interdental plaque (20%), persisting up to 3 months. However, a high proportion (50%) of all interdental sites were relatively unaffected by the different treatment modalities (Twetman and

Petersson 1997). According to Emilson (1994) the most persistent reduction of mutans streptococci has been achieved by varnishes, followed by gels and mouth rinses. However, as far as caries inhibition is concerned, a meta-analysis of different studies showed that neither the type of application nor the application frequency, caries risk, simultaneous fluoride regime, caries diagnosis, or tooth surface had any significant influence on the resulting effect (van Rijkom et al 1996).

If the gel is applied at home with a tray or a toothbrush, compliance of the patient is uncontrollable. A possible alternative to the "drastic" chlorhexidine gel treatment may be the use of a custom splint lined with 3% chlorhexidine citrate in an ethyl cellulose polymer. Such splints are worn nightly for 1 week. The procedure has reduced S mutans in the saliva for at least 3 months (Hildebrandt et al 1992).

OTHER ANTIPLAQUE PREPARATIONS

Phenolic compounds

Preparations containing phenolic compounds in the form of gargles and lozenges have long been used in treatment of throat and pharynx infections. They are said to have an antiplaque effect as well. Listerine contains 0.06% thymol, 0.09% oil of eucalyptus, 0.04% menthol, and 0.06% methyl salicylate. Aside from chlorhexidine, Listerine and comparable products are the only products recognized by the American Dental Association as reducing supragingival plaque and gingivitis significantly in comparison to a placebo. One study (DePaola et al 1989) indicated that plaque and gingivitis were reduced by

34% on average compared with a control group after use of Listerine for 6 months. However, the plaque-inhibitory effect of Listerine is lower than that provided by chlorhexidine (Axelsson and Lindhe 1987, Brecx et al 1990, Overholser et al 1990). The plaque-inhibitory effect of Listerine is increased through the use of a Water-pik (Ciancio et al 1989). Whether the plaque-inhibitory effect lasts sufficiently long to prevent the development of periodontitis remains an open question.

Sanguinaria

Sanguinaria, a substance used for more than 100 years in homeopathy, was examined for antiplaque activity in the late 1980s. It is a plant alkaloid extracted from the root of the North American poppy *Sanguinaria canadensis*. The material owes its antimicrobial and inflammation-inhibiting properties to an amino group.

Toxicologically harmless (Schwartz 1986) sanguinaria is the active agent in some oral rinses and toothpastes. These rinses sometimes contain zinc chloride (Viadent or Periogard); the Canadian Oragard-2 contains cetyl pyridinium chloride. Toothpastes containing sanguinaria usually are fluoridated as well.

In a concentration of 15 µg/mL, sanguinaria produces a 50% reduction in glucose uptake by S mutans as it also acts against S sanguis and actinomycetes in vitro (Eisenberg et al 1985). After use, sanguinaria can be demonstrated for 2 hours at a minimal inhibitory concentration in the plaque. The substance does not affect the total microbial population negatively, however (Southard et al 1984, Dzink and Socransky 1985). Although sanguinaria has high affinity to plaque, the active form is released only sparingly into the saliva (Goodson 1989).

Questions have been raised about both the effectiveness and the low pH of sanguinaria (Balanyk 1990). Although the pH of Viadent has been raised from 3.2 to 4.5, Periogard still has a pH of 3.0. Both of these products are fluoridated. Repeated use of oral rinses with such a low pH may lead to erosions, particularly in patients with exposed root surfaces. It has been reported, however, that salivary pH returns to 7.0 within 5 minutes after rinsing with Viadent (pH 4.5) (Harper et al 1990).

The temporary decrease in pH also may explain the very irregular results of clinical studies of products containing sanguinaria. Balanyk (1990) concluded, in a critical review of the numerous short-term and rare long-term studies that deal with this substance, that sanguinaria has no enduring usefulness in the reduction of plaque and gingivitis.

The use of sanguinaria has been also examined in patients with fixed orthodontic appliances. Palcanis et al (1986), Miller et al (1988), and Hannah et al (1989) observed clear plaque- and gingivitis-reducing effects of the material in their 2- to 6-month studies. Oral rinses and toothpastes containing sanguinaria were used together in each of these studies. Such a combination therapy is said to show an additive or synergistic effect (Harper et al 1990). Sanguinaria is regarded to be especially effective when it reaches the sulcus. That can be achieved with a sanguinaria toothpaste and a sulcular toothbrush and with an oral rinse used in a syringe (Svanbom and Davison 1987). Before such combination therapies can be recommended, however, additional independent long-term studies with adequately selected subjects are needed to demonstrate the plaque-inhibiting effect.

Quaternary ammonium compounds

Quaternary ammonium compounds can reduce surface energy, be absorbed from negatively charged tooth surfaces, and destroy membranes. These properties explain their clinical effects. Although the compounds are absorbed quickly in high concentration from the tooth surface, they are released as quickly, leading to low permanence; the permanence is substantially lower than that of chlorhexidine (Bonesvoll and Gjermo 1978). Mucosal irritation is a frequently observed side effect of quaternary ammonium compounds.

Cetyl pyridinium chloride is the most frequently used quaternary ammonium compound. It was suggested as a plaque-inhibiting material as early as the 1960s (Sturzenberger and Leonard 1969). Commercial products include Scope, Cepacol, and Reach. Some of these products also contain fluoride, so that daily use ensures an adequate local fluoride concentration.

Clinical studies indicate that the good in vitro results are not consistently confirmed in vivo. Although Bonesvoll and Gjermo (1978) reported that four-times daily rinsing with a solution containing 0.08% cetyl pyridinium chloride achieves nearly the plaque-inhibiting effect of chlorhexidine, other authors contest this view (Mandel 1988). Also, the compounds do not enhance the effectiveness of ordinary fluoridated toothpastes (Addy and Moran 1989).

Triclosan compounds

Broad-spectrum antimicrobial agents have been studied as components of toothpaste for some years. Because nearly 100% of the population uses toothpaste, such preparations would provide a good means to support at-home oral hygiene over long periods. Triclosan, a disinfecting material that has been used in medicine for years, is one such substance compatible with toothpastes.

Clinical studies have shown that triclosan has a very limited plaque-inhibiting effect (Cummins 1991). Three strategies have been used to improve the clinical effect. Thus, triclosan has been combined with: 1) zinc citrate, another antimicrobial additive (Mentadent P); 2) sodium pyrophosphate, a calculus inhibitor (Crest Ultra Protection); and 3) Gantrez copolymer (Colgate Gum Protection). Each of these toothpastes also contains fluoride.

A 7-month double-blind study of 185 subjects showed that the triclosan-zinc citrate combination was superior in all ways to the other combinations (Svatun et al 1993). Compared with the control group, which used an ordinary fluoride toothpaste, triclosan–zinc citrate reduced supragingival plaque formation by 33%, gingival bleeding by 51%, and calculus formation by 67%. The two other combinations affected only gingival bleeding. The effect of the triclosan–zinc citrate combination was demonstrable in the entire dentition, even in the posterior region, which is difficult to clean; researchers found that 36% less plaque was formed posteriorly in the study group than in the control group.

Whether this toothpaste has an equally good effect in the complex oral milieu of orthodontic treatment remains to be determined.

Prebrushing rinses

With much marketing effort, an oral rinse appeared several years ago with the claim that it removed plaque even before toothbrushing began and was effective even where the toothbrush did not reach. The oral rinse, Plax, contains sodium benzoate, polysorbate 20, and sodium lauryl sulfate as significant ingredients. The last ingredient, a surfactant, is a component of many toothpastes. Plax is not an antibacterial agent; rather, it is a surface-active material said to loosen the plaque so that it is easier to remove later.

In clinical studies, Plax, whether used in uncontrolled home oral care or under controlled conditions, proved to be no more effective than water for plaque inhibition (Grossman 1988, Singh 1990). The 6-month study required by the American Dental Association also reached the conclusion that Plax is no better than a placebo in reducing plaque, gingivitis, or calculus (Lobene et al 1990). This was confirmed in a study involving patients with fixed orthodontic appliances (Pointier et al 1990).

Due to these negative results, the formulation of Plax has been changed in Europe. The new ingredients may be more suitable for reducing plaque formation. The clinician must, therefore, advise patients against purchase of this oral rinse. Patients who believe the promotional slogans claiming plaque reduction ("also effective where the toothbrush doesn't reach" and "tooth rinse fights plaque") may neglect their mechanical toothbrushing. An added factor is that Plax contains no fluoride. Plax is directly contraindicated for concurrent use with chlorhexidine, because sodium lauryl sulfate drastically reduces the antibacterial effects of chlorhexidine (Imfeld and Saxer 1990). Also noteworthy is the fact that large amounts of sodium are absorbed through the oral tissues, which can provide problems for patients on low-sodium diets (Wagner et al 1989).

ANTIBIOTICS

An oral or systemic antibiotic regimen is indicated for otherwise uncontrollable periodontal lesions (eg, rapidly progressive periodontitis or recurrent periodontal abscess) to eliminate specific pathogenic organisms. Antibiotics always should be given in high doses for short periods (1 to 2 weeks). However, antibiotic therapy can never replace the mechanical removal of subgingival deposits; rather, it is a supplemental, supportive therapy (see review by Slots and Rams 1990).

As a result of the possible development of resistance when antibiotics are given systematically and the possible general side effects, local dosage forms providing longer release of the active form are now in the active phase of testing. For example, tetracycline fibers have been placed in recurring periodontal pockets (Addy et al 1988). These fibers release tetracycline continuously for 10 days and then are removed. To overcome the clinical difficulties of placing and removing the fibers, resorbable polymers containing doxycycline have been developed (Genco 1994). Recent findings indicate that tetracycline not only has an excellent antibiotic effect but also simultaneously inhibits the collagenase responsible for degradation of periodontal fibers. Furthermore, tetracycline has an anti-inflammatory effect; it inhibits bone resorption and is able to stimulate the attachment of fibroblasts to root surfaces (Seymour and Heasman 1995). Other slow-release drugs comprise metronidazole and minocycline (Genco 1994). Data presented so far have mostly shown reduced inflammation, while the effect upon the progression of the disease remains somewhat unknown (Gjermo 1993). However, these substances may be promising adjuncts to the treatment of recurrent periodontal lesions and early-onset periodontitis.

Antibiotic therapy, like the treatment of serious periodontal disease, belongs in the hands of an experienced specialist and should not be administered by an orthodontist.

CONCLUSIONS

Although plaque-inhibiting preparations for local application support oral hygiene and significantly decrease the risk of caries and periodontal disease, the clinician must not rely solely on their effects. Chemical substances that have only an antimicrobial effect, reduce the adhesion of bacteria to tooth surfaces, or modify plaque structure are, in the final analysis, only supplements to the elimination of plaque. Mechanical removal of plaque remains indispensable and is the basis for all preventive efforts.

Antimicrobial rinses are effective only on visible surfaces. They do not diffuse into interdental spaces to reduce plaque and inflammation at those sites (Finkelstein et al 1990). That can be achieved only with dental floss or tape. At present, chlorhexidine is the most potent gingivitis- and caries-reducing medicament. It should be used particularly by patients with a high risk of caries and by those with oral disease conditions not otherwise amenable to treatment. Although the danger of development of resistant bacterial strains does not appear particularly high, use of chlorhexidine solutions and gels always should be limited to brief periods. This limitation does not apply to varnishes, which offer the advantage of reservoir formation and continuous release of chlorhexidine.

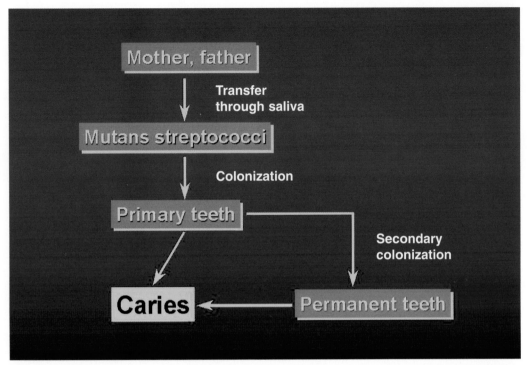

Fig 5-8 Infectious path of mutans streptococci from the parents to the primary and the permanent teeth of the child. In the end, this infection can lead to caries.

Chlorhexidine now is used successfully in pregnant and nursing women to interrupt the chain of infection by mutans streptococci. Because mothers with high levels of mutans streptococci can transfer this organism to their infants (Fig 5-8) (Köhler and Bratthall 1978), strict mechanical and chemical preventive measures should be used in an attempt to eliminate or reduce the levels in mothers. The results of these efforts have been surprisingly good. All subsequently born children have lower mutans streptococci values and caries is largely absent (Köhler et al 1983, Köhler et al 1984).

Systematic Program for Preventing Caries and Periodontal Disease in Orthodontic Patients

6

PATIENTS WITH REMOVABLE APPLIANCES

In comparison to partial or complete dentures, removable orthodontic appliances frequently provide more retention niches for bacterial deposits. The goal of oral hygiene must be the elimination of plaque in the oral cavity and on the appliances to prevent reinfection of the cleaned tooth surfaces.

One of two procedures is usually recommended to the patient for home care of removable appliances:

1. Cleaning with a toothbrush (and toothpaste or soap) under running water

2. Cleaning in a water bath containing a cleanser tablet

In a scanning electron microscopic study, Diedrich (1989) found appliances to be free of plaque if they were cleaned twice daily by the latter procedure. Even retention niches, such as resin under protrusion springs or screw spindles, were practically free of plaque. According to his observations, the combination of toothbrush and toothpaste cleaned only the easily accessible surfaces of the appliances adequately. However, the use of self-acting cleansing tablets cannot be recommended without reservation. According to Rabe et al (1987), between 2% and 3% of total deposits remain on the appliances being cleaned. Furthermore, the antibacterial effectiveness of such tablet cleansers is doubtful, and they lead to obvious corrosion of the silver solder connections (Rabe et al 1986).

One convincing explanation for the contradictory results might be that the tablet cleansers are highly effective only they are used regularly from the very first day. However, once a plaque film has developed—and presumably that is the case very often—the use of such cleanser tablets alone does not result in a thorough cleaning of removable appliances.

Almost unlimited removal of microorganisms, in contrast, occurs when orthodontic appliances are cleaned in an ultrasonic bath (eg, Ultraclin). However, this method is associated with significant costs for the patient (Diedrich 1989). One possible compromise is the ultrasonic cleaning of the devices at each treatment appointment. This effective type of cleaning also is useful for breaking the potential patient–dental laboratory–patient chain of infection when an appliance requires repair.

It is very difficult to keep removable appliances completely free of plaque.

Consequently, it seems logical to inhibit the deposition of plaque on such devices and the adjoining tooth surfaces with chlorhexidine. A recently developed preparation, SRD (slow-release dosage) chlorhexidine, is interesting in this regard. After application, it releases its active ingredient on the surface of the appliance for approximately 1 week without leading to tooth discoloration or alteration of taste. The plaque-reducing effect of the product has been demonstrated microbiologically and clinically (Friedman et al 1985, Zyskind et al 1990). That material is not commercially available at present. However, commercially available chlorhexidine varnishes (eg, Cervitec) that are applied on the surface of the PMMA may be used instead. Cervitec successfully reduced cariogenic bacteria like mutans streptococci on cervical (Huizinga et al 1990) and proximal surfaces (Petersson et al 1991) and prevented or healed primary root carious lesions (Lynch and Beighton 1994). For reducing interdental bacteria, three applications within 2 weeks are more effective than monthly applications for 3 months (Twetman and Petersson 1997).

A polymethyl methacrylate resin that releases fluoride (Orthocryl Plus) is being marketed. Its slow release of fluoride over a period of many months provides an enduring, low concentration of fluoride in the saliva. This release of fluoride provides good conditions for the remineralization of initial mineralization defects (Miethke and Newesely 1987, 1988, Alaçam et al 1996).

PATIENTS WITH FIXED APPLIANCES

Ideally, orthodontic treatment is a caries-preventive measure in itself (Feliu 1982). It

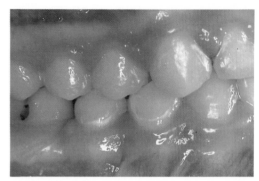

Fig 6-1 Garland-shaped cervical zones of demineralization are present on the maxillary right lateral incisor and canine and the mandibular right premolars after bracket removal. The hyperplastic papillae are an expression of poor oral hygiene.

is probably the experience of every orthodontist, however, that massive initial lesions and sometimes more advanced enamel destruction are found when bands and brackets are removed (Fig 6-1). Systematic caries-preventive care is the only sensible means for the avoidance of such conditions.

Phases of prophylaxis

The literature provides many suggestions for preventive programs for patients with fixed appliances (Zachrisson 1974, Zachrisson 1975, Clark 1976, Shannon 1981, Dénes et al 1986, Yeung et al 1989, Berglund and Small 1990). But prevention naturally begins long before the actual orthodontic therapy, in the consultation and planning phase. According to Lundström et al (1980) and Hotz (1982), three phases of prophylaxis can be defined in this connection:

1. Preventive measures before treatment:
   a. Motivation
   b. Oral hygiene training

c. Professional tooth cleaning
d. Diet counseling
2. Preventive measures during active treatment:
   a. Control of oral hygiene
   b. Fluoride application
   c. Diet counseling
   d. Chemical plaque control
3. Preventive measures during retention:
   a. Control of oral hygiene
   b. Fluoride application
   c. Remineralization
   d. Diet counseling

The greatest danger to dental hard tissue and the periodontium arises in the first 4 months after placement of fixed appliances. Even with good oral hygiene practice on the part of the patient, plaque deposition and symptoms of gingivitis increase, although they decrease thereafter (Lundström et al 1980, Pender 1986). Therefore, special attention must be paid during this period.

Simplified preventive concept

Although the phase distinction described above appears logical and sensible, it is not advisable to be oriented only to the treatment phase. In practice, almost all preventive measures arise during all treatment phases, and they should be weighed more or less equally. A simplified preventive concept consisting of the following steps in three phases appears to be more suitable.

1. Basic prevention:
   a. Oral hygiene with fluoridated toothpaste, dental floss, and/or interdental brushes
   b. Professional tooth cleaning
   c. Fluoride rinses
   d. Fluoride varnish on high-risk surfaces (four times yearly)

e. Diet counseling
2. Supplementary prevention:
   a. Chemical plaque control
      1. Chlorhexidine gel in custom trays
      2. Chlorhexidine varnish on high-risk surfaces (four times yearly)
3. Recall:
   a. Professional tooth cleaning
   b. Remotivation and reinstruction
   c. Evaluation for additional preventive measures

This concept not only relates to patients with fixed appliances, but also can be applied generally. Every patient should practice basic prevention. If basic prevention is insufficient or special caries- or periodontitis-promoting factors are present, additional preventive measures must be implemented. All of these considerations must be evaluated at regular recall appointments.

To reduce the damage to dental hard tissue and the periodontium to a minimum during orthodontic treatment, the following prerequisites must be fulfilled from the very beginning:

1. Low risk of periodontitis
2. Low risk of caries
3. Treatment of all carious lesions
4. Patient instruction and motivation
5. Efficient recall system

If these conditions are not provided, orthodontic treatment should not even be initiated. If the oral hygiene of a patient deteriorates, for any reason at all, during treatment, or if significant periodontal destruction develops, the orthodontist must have the courage to interrupt or to discontinue the treatment. Unavoidable demineralization, carious lesions, and tooth loss can devastate all orthodontic efforts.

113

A patient thus affected may well demand—not without cause—compensation for irreversible tooth defects.

Risk of periodontitis

Little evidence exists that orthodontic treatment increases the risk of later development of periodontal disease. Various studies have compared patient groups treated 10 to 35 years earlier with fixed orthodontic appliances with untreated control groups and have concluded that almost no differences exist (Sadowsky and BeGole 1981, Polson and Reed 1984). Nevertheless, if adult patients with existing periodontal disease are treated orthodontically, it must be assured that the periodontal condition remains under control through root scaling, root planing, and excellent oral hygiene practice (Rateitschak 1968). In such instances it is desirable to work with a periodontist, so that possible periodontal complications can be avoided from the outset (Figs 6-2a and 6-2b).

Orthodontic therapy following periodontal treatment need not injure the periodontium, provided that effective oral hygiene and follow-up care are provided (Ramfjord 1985). Rapid periodontal destruction is programmed if these require-

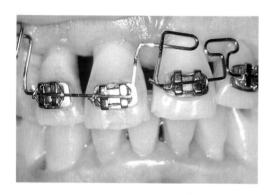

Fig 6-2a and 6-2b Generalized horizontal bone resorption is present. Orthodontic tooth movement is possible even in patients with advanced periodontal disease, if light, directional forces are used. An inflammation-free periodontium is the prerequisite that can be achieved only through periodontal therapy and a rigorous recall system.

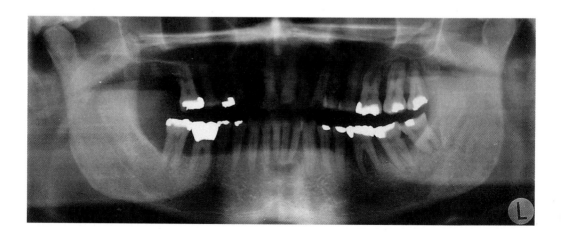

ments are not met. If orthodontic treatment is attempted in the presence of inflamed periodontal tissue, supragingival plaque may be displaced subgingivally, leading to loss of attachment (Ericsson et al 1977).

Some authors recommend that at least 6 months be allowed for healing of the involved tissues after subgingival scaling before orthodontic treatment is initiated (Baderstein et al 1984b). In principle, that means a hygiene phase of 4 to 6 months before active orthodontic therapy (Eliasson et al 1982). If guided tissue regeneration has been provided, at least 6 months should elapse between the time the membrane is removed and orthodontic treatment is begun (Kokich and Mathews 1989).

If periodontal health of a patient is established and assured for the longer term, tooth movement leads to practically no loss of attachment, even when the attachment is already seriously reduced. All tooth movement should be done bodily and preferably intrusively (Miethke and Melsen 1993). If a reduced periodontium is inflamed, however, orthodontic treatment can lead quickly to tooth loss (Boyd et al 1989).

The orthodontist mostly deals with adult patients who have slowly progressive (adult) periodontitis. Such a condition develops from gingivitis between age 30 and 40, and accounts for 95% of all periodontal diseases. Molars are affected most frequently, followed by anterior teeth. Bone loss associated with this form of periodontitis initially is horizontal, usually with occurrence of periodontal pockets. Later, vertical loss occurs, accompanied by bone pockets.

Only approximately 5% of all periodontal disease is of the rapidly progressive type that begins in the third decade of life and affects women in particular. The severity and course of this disease vary greatly, but acute episodes with sometimes deep vertical bone pockets always are caused by specific microorganisms. In general, patients with rapidly progressive periodontitis should be excluded from orthodontic therapy.

Localized juvenile periodontitis, characterized by significant, rapid bone loss in the region of the incisors and first molars, poses a significant risk to successful orthodontic therapy (Baer and Everett 1975). Fortunately, this condition accounts for only approximately 0.1% of all periodontal diseases; girls are affected three times more frequently than boys. Because localized juvenile periodontitis develops during puberty, the orthodontist may be the first to identify the condition.

Although periodontal problems arise infrequently or not at all in children and adolescents (Zachrisson and Alnæs 1973, Alstad and Zachrisson 1979), the orthodontist must recognize the development of periodontal lesions quickly and take steps to eliminate them. Gingival hyperplasia is a frequent problem seen not only when lingual appliances are used. The condition occurs predominantly in the anterior region, particularly in the mandible. Figures 6-3a to 6-3d show extensive gingival hyperplasia affecting all maxillary anterior teeth of an 11-year-old boy. Bleeding was easily provoked by light probing with a periodontal probe, an indication of acute periodontitis. Despite professional cleaning at 2-week intervals and use of chlorhexidine, no improvement occurred. For that patient, gingivectomy was required to provide adequate oral hygiene conditions that further could be controlled by the patient.

The bleeding tendency of the periodontium should be determined routinely with a periodontal probe, and probing

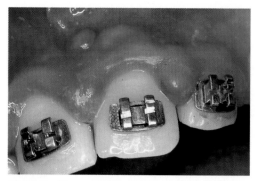

Fig 6-3a The maxillary incisors of an 11-year-old boy exhibit gingival hyperplasia.

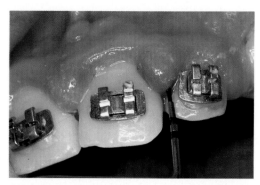

Fig 6-3b Gingival probing between the left central and lateral incisors shows a 5.0-mm pocket.

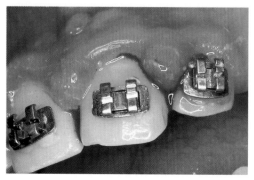

Fig 6-3c Profuse interdental hemorrhage indicates severe inflammation of the marginal periodontium.

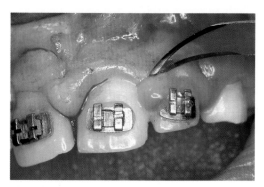

Fig 6-3d Gingivectomy is required to allow adequate oral hygiene.

depth should be measured to determine gingival and periodontal problems early (Haffajee et al 1983). A bleeding periodontium is always associated with an inflammatory process and deserves special attention.

Guidelines for the orthodontic treatment of adolescents and adults with periodontal lesions are provided in Box 6-1. Joint treatment with a periodontist often is advisable for such patients.

Systematic caries risk evaluation and preventive/therapeutic consequences

The question of whether additional laboratory analyses are required to determine a patient's risk of caries is decided on the basis of the subject's caries experience and the existing clinical caries activity. Targeted preventive and therapeutic measures are initiated in accordance with the diagnosis, which also establishes the recall intervals. A diagnosis, once established, is not necessarily final; it must be confirmed or corrected at regular intervals. A relatively low risk for caries can change quickly to a high risk if the attack mechanism–defense reaction relationship is altered suddenly.

An assessment of caries risk must be made at a safe time span before orthodontic treatment, preferably during the ini-

Box 6-1 Guidelines for Orthodontic Treatment of Patients with Periodontal Lesions

Examination

Probing of the gingival sulcus

No bleeding: Healthy periodontium
Minimal bleeding: Minor inflammation—Requires further observation
Immediate, heavy bleeding: Active inflammation—Requires treatment (see below)

Measurement of sulcular probing depth

1 – 3 mm: Physiologic
3 – 4 mm: Minor periodontal damage—Requires intensification of oral hygiene measures
> 4 mm: Significant periodontal damage—Requires treatment

Therapy

Before orthodontic treatment

1. Hygiene phase:
   a. Oral hygiene instruction and motivation
2. Periodontal therapy (initial):
   a. in adult periodontitis, subgingival scaling when pockets are present
   b. in rapidly progressive periodontitis, subgingival scaling 6 months before treatment
3. Periodontal treatment (consecutive):
   a. in rapidly progressive periodontitis with actively inflamed periodontal lesions, local treatment with tetracycline and/or flap surgery

During orthodontic treatment

1. Oral hygiene instruction and motivation
2. Periodontal examination:
   a. in adult periodontitis and rapidly progressive periodontitis, professional tooth cleaning approximately every 3 months
   b. in rapidly progressive periodontitis, deep scaling of bleeding periodontal pockets
   c. in rapidly progressive periodontitis, deep scaling before and after active intrusion

After orthodontic treatment

1. In adult periodontitis and rapidly progressive periodontitis, deep scaling after removal of orthodontic attachments
2. Oral hygiene instruction and motivation:
   a. reinstruction to avoid gingival recessions and wedge-shaped defects

Patients at high risk during orthodontic treatment

1. Patients with adult periodontitis or rapidly progressive periodontitis who have poor oral hygiene
2. Patients with rapidly progressive periodontitis who have recurring deep pockets
3. Patients with adult periodontitis or rapidly progressive periodontitis who have furcation defects
4. Patients with localized juvenile periodontitis

tial diagnosis. In this way, the orthodontist gains sufficient time to initiate appropriate prophylactic measures. Thereafter, it is necessary to ascertain that the risk of caries remains at a low level during active orthodontic treatment.

An appropriate prevention strategy, according to our experience, is described on the basis of three examples below. The program is depicted graphically in Figs 6-4a and 6-4b.

Patients with clinically high carious activity. High caries activity is characterized clinically by teeth that are obviously carious or bitewing radiographs that show carious demineralization. The color and low hardness of clinical lesions indicate that they will progress (Figs 6-5a and 6-5b). Mutans streptococci and lactobacilli tests provide no additional evidence here; they would serve only to confirm the clinical diagnosis, document it, and demonstrate the problem to the patient.

The first step in treatment of such patients is the removal of all microbial deposits. The patient must be made conscious of oral hygiene. Explanations of the cause of dental disease, instruction for home care, and diet counseling follow. This sequence holds for all patients.

The second step is treatment, at least provisionally, of all carious lesions and, in adolescents, application of pit and fissure sealant if needed. Similarly, secondary caries must be restored and overhanging margins corrected. In this way, niches in which mutans streptococci and lactobacilli can proliferate are eliminated. If chlorhexidine were applied alone, rapid reinfection with mutans streptococci could occur. Mutans streptococci present in carious depressions and fissures are not necessarily reached by agents that act locally; such agents attack only organisms on smooth

surfaces. Mutans streptococci continue to proliferate in those niches that continue to exist and infect smooth surfaces. Initial carious lesions are not restored but are remineralized with a fluoride varnish or oral rinses containing fluoride.

Premolar fissures usually are not very deep and complex in shape and therefore only rarely require sealant application. Teeth in their eruptive phase cannot be sealed immediately. It is desirable to protect the occlusal surfaces that are still partly covered by mucosa with chlorhexidine or fluoride varnish. Later application of sealant may be superfluous, especially if the caries risk is changed to low, the morphology of the fissures limits plaque retention, or if both conditions exist.

Sealants should be applied only until 6 years following eruption, however. That is the period of greatest danger of caries. In adults, pits and fissures should be treated with a chlorhexidine varnish, instead.

The third step in treatment is antimicrobial therapy with chlorhexidine. Chlorhexidine gel, applied via soft custom trays, is preferable to a rinse solution, because the gel remains in contact with the teeth for longer periods. It is important that chlorhexidine be applied in a concentrated form over a defined period. Two procedures have proven valuable for the purpose: The patient may apply the chlorhexidine once daily at home for 2 weeks. Alternatively, if the cooperation required of the patient or his or her parents is questionable, an intensive application of chlorhexidine can be made in the dental office over 2 consecutive days. These procedures are described in more detail in chapter 5.

The mutans streptococci titer can be reduced significantly and quickly through these procedures. Without further treatment, new inoculation occurs only after 2

Figs 6-4a and 6-4b Summary of the prophylaxis concept described in the text. The upper portions are identical; the lower portions have been separated to provide clarity. OH = oral hygiene; CR = caries risk. + = good; − = poor; ⇑ = high; ⇓ = low.

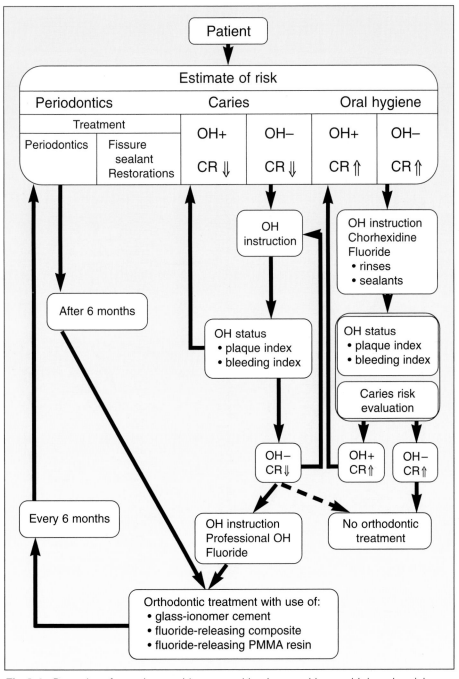

Fig 6-4a Procedure for patients with poor oral hygiene and low or high caries risk.

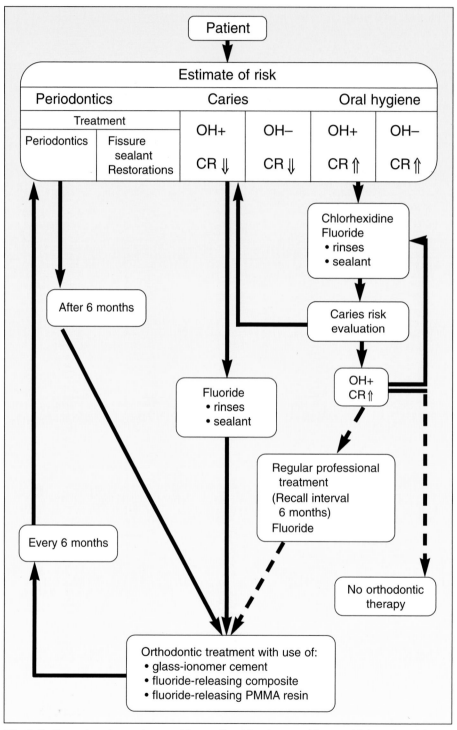

Fig 6-4b Procedure for patients with good oral hygiene and low or high caries risk.

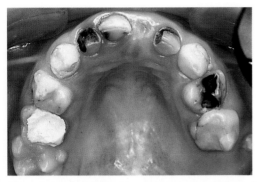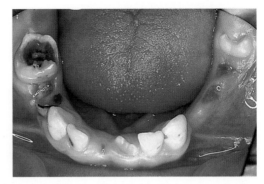

Figs 6-5a and 6-5b Numerous open carious lesions are present. The caries activity and future caries risk is obviously high in this patient. Salivary microorganism tests are superfluous, because they would only confirm the clinical impression.

to 3 months. This provides sufficient time to complete definitive restorative treatment and to eliminate the ecological niches for cariogenic organisms through oral hygiene instruction, diet counseling, and fluoridation measures.

Such chlorhexidine therapy should be provided in its entirety. Though mutans streptococci do not adhere to the plastic rods of the Dentocult SM strip after a single application of the gel, these bacteria nevertheless can be cultured from saliva in the laboratory. To determine the actual results of chlorhexidine treatment, a Dentocult SM strip test should be performed no earlier than 2 weeks after therapy has ended.

Patients with restorations but assumed clinically low carious activity. Restorations always reflect some caries experience because, as a rule, a carious lesion was the reason for the restoration. However, no reliable reference point exists initially for determining the patient's risk of caries (Figs 6-6a and 6-6b). Existing restorations indicate that high caries activity was present in the past, but it is not known if the factors causing caries exist

currently and will in the future. As a result, the clinician faces a dilemma.

Microbiologic studies, however, provide information about possible sources of attack. In these patients, therefore, immediate estimation of mutans streptococci and lactobacilli is in order. If the mutans streptococci count is high, the chlorhexidine procedures described earlier are followed. If the count is low, the resistance of the tooth surfaces must be increased by application of fluoride.

Patients with a caries-free dentition. In a caries-free dentition (which means no evidence of caries in bitewing radiographs either), the probability is great that the risk of caries actually is low (Figs 6-7a and 6-7b). This decision should be made in consideration of the patient's age as well. The caries-free dentition of a 10-year-old child must be evaluated differently than that of a 20-year-old individual. The child still is in the period of the mixed dentition, and 12 to 16 teeth are in eruption or will erupt in the next 2 to 3 years. Attack factors can change quickly during this time. In the 20-year-old, in contrast, the balance in favor of resistance factors would appear to be

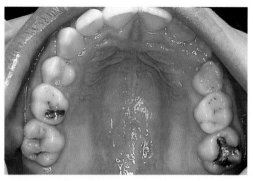
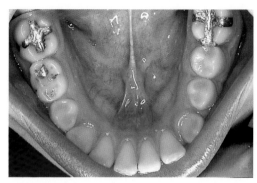

Figs 6-6a and 6-6b Oral hygiene is good, but several restorations are present, indicating past caries activity. The purely clinical evaluation in such instances is problematic, so an assessment of salivary microorganism levels is indicated.

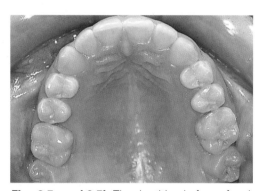
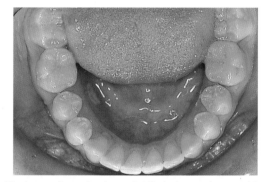

Figs 6-7a and 6-7b The dentition is free of caries. To determine whether a labile balance that could be altered toward the development of caries by the placement of a fixed appliance exists in this young patient, microbial salivary analysis should be performed.

well established. Secondary maturation of the surface enamel is complete; furthermore, the teeth have found their positions in the jaws and no changes are to be anticipated in the interproximal spaces.

Nevertheless, the conditions may change in both instances. Changes in diet or a severe disease can lead to an increase in caries-causing agents, preparing the way for an attack on the hard tissue. The consequences may not be clinically apparent until 1 or 2 years later. For that

reason, examination of saliva of caries-free patients is not necessary routinely but is helpful in establishing the clinical diagnosis.

Principles of optimal orthodontic treatment in relation to oral hygiene

The following preventive measures should be fulfilled for optimal orthodontic treatment regarding caries and periodontal disease prevention:

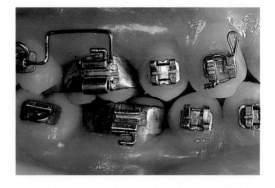

Fig 6-8 The molar bands have been shortened, for reasons of periodontal prophylaxis, to the extent that they are clearly supragingival in the buccal regions.

1. The need for an orthodontic attachment must be evaluated separately for each tooth; not everything that is white must be given an orthodontic band. Brackets are preferable to bands for periodontal reasons.

2. Orthodontic bands should be shortened so that their gingival margins are positioned supragingivally (Fig 6-8).

3. To prevent demineralization around the bracket bases, fluoride-releasing adhesives are preferred and fluoride varnish should be applied immediately after bracket placement and at 3-month intervals thereafter.

4. In general, glass-ionomer cements are preferable for orthodontic bands to prevent demineralization.

5. Excess adhesive and cement remnants should be eliminated for caries- and periodontal prophylaxis reasons.

6. The adhesion of all attachments must be checked regularly; loose bands and brackets must be recemented/re-bonded immediately.

7. Labial tipping especially of mandibular front teeth must be avoided if the gingiva propria is narrow and thin. A free gingival graft may be considered.

8. Retainers should be designed so that they interfere as little as possible with oral hygiene. Removable retention devices must be easy for the patient to clean; if they are constructed of polymethyl methacrylate resin, a fluoride-releasing material should be used.

Motivation and instruction

Motivation and instruction often are mere slogans. It is so difficult to enlist the cooperation of patients in ordinary practice that optimal motivation and instruction rarely happens. *Motivation* signifies an influence toward healthy nutrition. It must be made clear to a patient and his or her parents that a healthy, varied diet that contains as little sugar (sucrose) as possible is not only good for the teeth, but also a positive factor for the development of the patient as a whole. Of course, it is very difficult to prove that this recommendation is followed. As already noted, it is possible to check claims of patients (and their parents) indirectly with the lactobacillus test (see chapter 3).

Instruction relates to development of good oral hygiene practice. The orthodontist/dentist and specially trained personnel require much time to sensitize a patient to

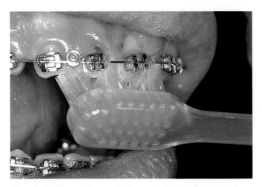

Fig 6-9 Cleansing of the tooth surfaces coronally and cervically of an orthodontic archwire with a conventional toothbrush.

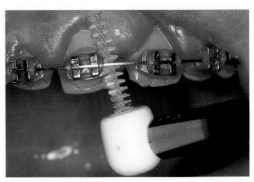

Fig 6-10 Effective cleansing of the tooth surfaces on the sides of the base of the bracket with an interdental brush.

his or her oral hygiene. A patient undergoing fixed appliance therapy must make special efforts with his or her teeth, because tooth cleaning is made significantly more difficult. The ortho-plaque-index and the gingival bleeding index are recommended for purposes of documentation and motivation of the patient.

The patient should use a normal toothbrush with a flat bristle field and a short head; special orthodontic toothbrushes have no advantages (Fig 6-9). Devices such as Superfloss and interdental brushes must be used by the patient to clean not only the proximal surfaces but also the tooth surfaces around brackets (Fig 6-10) and band margins. The patient may be instructed in the modified Bass technique (short, circular, vibrating movements, with a 45-degree angle between brush and tooth surface) because this provides better cleaning than the scrubbing method (back and forth movement of the brush). Despite its advantages, the Bass technique should not be elevated to the

status of dogma. Adequate cleaning of proximal surfaces is only possible with dental floss.

Newer electrically powered toothbrushes (Interplak, Rota-Dent, plaque remover) can simplify tooth cleaning and make it more acceptable. The Water-Pik device is effective only in combination with pharmaceutical adjuvants such as chlorhexidine or Listerine, if at all.

Perfect tooth cleaning requires at least 10 minutes for patients with fixed appliances, something the patient should be told before therapy begins. Motivation for oral hygiene that intensive must be reinforced regularly; such reinforcement is impossible without a recall system. In practice, that means planning time for a recall session for every third or fourth orthodontic treatment appointment.

Recall

The intervals between recalls depend on the caries risk determined initially; they vary between 1 month and 4 months. A recall examination during the active orthodontic treatment and retention phases should include the following:

1. Determination of the caries risk (eg, mutans streptococci, lactobacilli)
2. Determination of the degree of inflammation of the gingiva (periodontitis risk)
3. Professional tooth cleaning
4. Application of a fluoride varnish around bracket bases and on initial caries lesions

Interpretation of the number of bacteria present is difficult once multiband therapy has begun, because the numbers of caries-relevant bacteria always increase because of the artificial retention sites. It is alarming, however, when the number of mutans streptococci reaches the level of 500,000 to 1,000,000 colony-forming units. If such levels are found, temporary intervention with chlorhexidine is indicated (Fig 6-11). Chlorhexidine oral rinses also should be prescribed for a short period if the degree of inflammation of the gingiva is increased.

Plaque retention cervical to the bracket base and under a band can lead to demineralization in patients with fixed orthodontic appliances. Even 5 years after orthodontic treatment, the appearance of initial lesions may be significantly higher among former patients than in a comparable but not orthodontically treated control group, as demonstrated in a study by Øgaard (1989). The mandibular canines and premolars and the maxillary lateral incisors appeared to be especially susceptible.

Demineralization is best prevented by the strategically sound use of fluorides. Application of fluorides should accompany all preventive and treatment steps. But it is not enough to have the patient rinse daily with a fluoride preparation. Because of the existing retention elements, such a rinse does not reach all of the surfaces at risk sufficiently, and the rinse itself is quickly eliminated by the saliva. Poor cooperation on the part of the patient may also lessen the success.

For these reasons, it is desirable that the orthodontist/dentist or the dental hygienist treat the at-risk surfaces with a fluoride varnish at regular intervals. That should be done immediately after placement of the orthodontic attachments, during active therapy at 3-month intervals, and immediately after removal of all fixed appliances.

An orthodontic retainer should have caries-preventive effects and be designed so that cleaning is easy and that it does not cause any damage over the long term (Fig 6-12). For these reasons, removable retainers are preferable to fixed ones. The retainers should be as small as conditions permit so that they interfere with natural cleaning of the teeth as little as possible. Furthermore, the material used to fabricate the retainer should have a caries-inhibiting effect through the release of fluoride. An advantage of removable devices is that they can be used additionally as carriers of medicaments for intensive prophylaxis.

Increased plaque and calculus accumulation may be anticipated along the wires and on and around the resin composite adhesive when adhesively attached retainers, eg, a 3-3 lingual retainer, are used (Zachrisson 1977). Nevertheless, fixed retainers are said to lead to no initial lesions or periodontal damage when properly fabricated (Årtun 1984), even when they have been in situ for 2 years (Gorelick et al 1982). The type of wire used, smooth or stranded, has no role in this (Årtun 1984). Of course, a regular recall program should also be maintained during the retention phase.

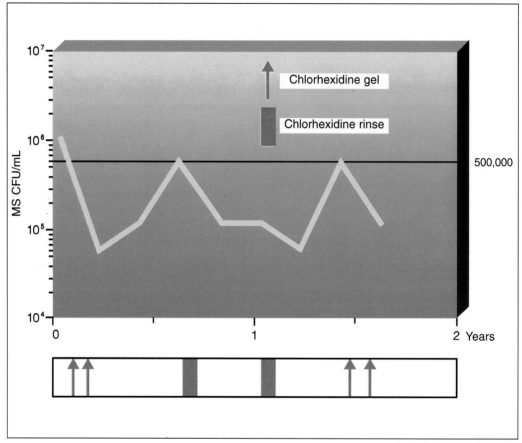

Fig 6-11 A schematic representation of chlorhexidine intervention in relation to the *S mutans* count during a 2-year orthodontic treatment period: a 14-year old boy has an *S mutans* value of 10^6 CFU/mL saliva at the beginning of treatment. After an intensive chlorhexidine regimen, the count sinks to 5×10^4 CFU/mL. During the active orthodontic treatment, the *S mutans* count again climbs quickly and after 4 months reaches a value of 5×10^5 CFU/mL saliva. Rinsing with chlorhexidine for 2 to 3 weeks causes the *S mutans* value to sink again. After approximately 1½ years the *S mutans* value begins to climb again, necessitating further chlorhexidine treatment. Intermittent chlorhexidine rinses prolong the reduction in bacteria.

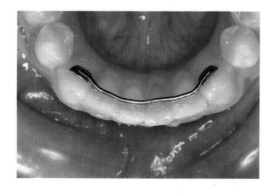

Fig 6-12 An adhesively fastened lingual retainer that can easily be cleaned with a toothbrush and Superfloss.

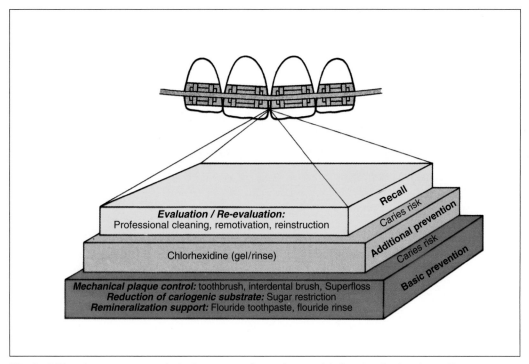

Fig 6-13 The three-stage prophylaxis concept for patients with fixed orthodontic appliances.

CONCLUSIONS

To plan successful orthodontic therapy, the practitioner must understand its risks for the hard tissue and the tooth-supporting tissue. The dangers arising from poor oral hygiene are obvious. Subsequent damage can be avoided only through continuous evaluation of these risks and targeted preventive and therapeutic measures. Naturally, the patient bears the responsibility for his or her dentition. But the orthodontist/dentist must retain control, must instruct, and must provide guidance. It is not prudent to apply prevention to each patient in the exact same way. It is the art of the clinician, based on his or her knowledge and experience, to select the preventive means appropriate for each patient. Certain principles, summarized in Fig 6-13, are important to this process.

Because patients with orthodontic appliances, particularly fixed appliances, require special care in terms of the prevention of caries and gingivitis, orthodontists are afforded a special opportunity for training these individuals for enduring oral health. That training can have positive effects long after the period of orthodontic treatment (Davies et al 1991).

Oral health is not a coincidence. It is a specific task of the orthodontist/dentist and of the auxiliary personnel to provide the best possible concept of prevention on that basis. In that way, the clinician can exert a significant influence on the healthy development of the dentition during the delicate mixed-dentition stage. That does not imply that every patient must be trained to be an obedient toothbrush acrobat, a sugar abstainer, or a hygiene perfectionist (Hotz 1982). It is important to sensitize the patient to the ecosystem of the mouth, to awaken his or her interest in oral health, and to impart the appropriate caries and gingivitis prophylaxis.

Carefully refined preventive schemes do not have the deciding role here; rather, it is the individual appraisal of each patient for risk of caries, gingivitis, and periodontitis. This can be determined relatively well through precise diagnosis and microbiologic tests. Depending on the existing risk, basic preventive measures must be supplemented by other means. The therapeutic use of fluorides is important for support of remineralization, as are the limitation of sugar intake to main meals and guidance toward effective oral hy-

giene. Individually adjusted recall appointments are crucial so that the patient can be remotivated and reinstructed. For all these efforts, the dentist and the orthodontist should be able to rely on trained personnel to take on some of the comprehensive work involved. Without the efforts of dental hygienists, a high-standard preventive program cannot be provided over the long term.

Every preventive concept that takes these principles into consideration and follows them can be a practical one. If it takes place within the framework of orthodontic treatment, it will contribute greatly to oral health.

References

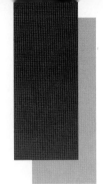

Abelson DC, Barton JE, Maietti GM, Cowherd MG. Evaluation of interproximal cleaning by two types of dental floss. J Clin Prev Dent 3:19–21, 1981.

Addy M, Hassan H, Moran J, Wade W, Newcombe R. Use of antimicrobial containing acurlic strips in the treatment of chronic periodontal disease. J Periodontol 59:557–564, 1988.

Addy M, Moran J. The effect of cetylpyridinium chloride (CPC) detergent foam compared to a conventional toothpaste on plaque and gingivitis. A single blind crossover study. J Clin Periodontol 16:87–91, 1989.

Adrianens ML, Dermout LR, Verbeeck RM. The use of Fluor, a fluoride varnish, as a caries prevention method under orthodontic molar bands. Eur J Orthod 12:316–319, 1990.

Ainamo J. Relationship between malalignment of the teeth and periodontal disease. Scan J Dent Res 80:104–110, 1972.

Ainamo J, Bay I. Problems and proposals for recording gingivitis and plaque. Int Dent J 25:229–235, 1975.

Ainamo J, Hormia M, Kaunaisaho K, Sorsa T, Soumalainen K. Klinische Studie zur Wirksamkeit des Plaque-Entferners Braun Plak Control (D 5) im Vergleich zu einer herkömmlichen elektrischen Zahnbürste (Braun D 3) und einer manuellen Zahnbürste. Manufacturer's information, Braun, Frankfurt, Germany, 1991.

Ainamo J, Xie Q, Ainamo A, Kallio P. Assessment of the effect of an oscillating/rotating electric toothbrush on oral health. A 12-month longitudinal study. J Clin Periodontol 24:28–33, 1997.

Alaçam A, Ulusu T, Bordur H, Öztas N, Ören MC. Salivary and urinary fluoride levels after 1-month use of fluoride-releasing removable appliances. Caries Res 30:200–203, 1996.

Alaluusua S, Kleemola-Kujala E, Nyström M, Evalahti M, Grönroos L. Caries in the primary teeth and salivary Streptococcus mutans and lactobacillus levels as indicators of caries in permanent teeth. Pediatr Dent 9:126–130, 1987.

Albandar JM. A 6-year study on the pattern of periodontal disease progression. J Clin Periodontol 17:467–471, 1990.

Alexander J. Toothbrushes and toothbrushing. In: Menaker L (ed). The Biological Basis of Dental Disease. Hagerstown, MD, Harper & Row, 457, 1980.

Alstad S, Zachrisson BU. Longitudinal study of periodontal condition associated with orthodontic treatment in adolescents. Am J Orthod 76: 277–286, 1979.

Anderman II. Pedodontic electrosurgery. J Pedod 14:202–213, 1989.

Andlin-Sobocki A, Marcussin A, Persson M. 3-year observation on gingival recession in mandibular incisors in children. J Clin Periodontol 18:155–159, 1991.

Angmar-Månsson B, Al-Khateeb S, Tranaeus S. Monitoring the caries process. Optical methods for clinical diagnosis and quantification of enamel caries. Eur J Oral Sci 104:480–485, 1996.

Arends J, Christoffersen J. Nature and role of loosely bound fluoride in dental caries. J Dent Res 69 (special issue):601–605, 1990.

Arends J, Duschner H, Ruben JL. Penetration of varnishes into demineralized root dentine in vitro. Caries Res 31:201–205, 1997.

129

Arends J, Schuthof J. Fluoride content in human enamel after fluoride application and washing. An in vitro study. Caries Res 9:363–372, 1975.

Armitage GC. Diagnostic tests for periodontal diseases. Curr Opin Dent 2:53–62, 1992.

Årtun J. Caries and periodontal reactions associated with long-term use of different types of bonded lingual retainers. Am J Orthod 86: 112–118, 1984.

Årtun J, Krogstad O. Periodontal status of mandibular incisors following excessive proclination. A study in adults with surgically treated mandibular prognathism. Am J Orthod 91: 225–232, 1987.

Ashley FP, Sainsbury RH. The effect of a school-based plaque control programme on caries and gingivitis. Br Dent J 150:41–45, 1981.

Atherton JD. The gingival response of orthodontic tooth movement. Am J Orthod 58:179–186, 1970.

Axelsson P. Salivary S mutans, Plaque Formation Rate Index PFRI and Cariostat-test in relation to caries prevalence in 14 year old children. Presented at The First International Conference on Preventive Dentistry and Epidemiology, Sunne, Sweden, 1988.

Axelsson P. Methode zur Bestimmung des Kariesrisikos. Phillip J 7:181–187, 1990.

Axelsson P. A four-point scale for selection of caries risk patients, based on salivary S. mutans levels and plaque formation rate index. In: Johnson N (ed): Risk Markers for Oral Diseases. London, Cambridge University Press, 158–170, 1991.

Axelsson P, Lindhe J. The effect of a preventive programme on dental plaque, gingivitis and caries in schoolchildren. Results after one and two years. J Clin Periodontol 1:126–138, 1974.

Axelsson P, Lindhe J. The effect of a plaque control program on gingivitis and dental caries in schoolchildren. J Dent Res 56:142–148, 1977.

Axelsson P, Lindhe J. Effect of controlled oral hygiene procedures on caries and periodontal disease in adults. Results after 6 years. J Clin Periodontol 8:239–248, 1981.

Axelsson P, Lindhe J. Efficacy of mouthrinses in inhibiting dental plaque and gingivitis in man. J Clin Periodontol 14:205–212, 1987.

Axelsson P, Lindhe J, Nyström B. On the prevention of caries and periodontal disease. Results of a 15-year longitudinal study in adults. J Clin Periodontol 18:182–189, 1991.

Axelsson P, Paulander J, Nordkvist K, Karlsson R. Effect of fluoride-containing dentifrice, mouthrinsing, and varnish on approximal dental caries in a 3-year clinical trial. Community Dent Oral Epidemiol 15:177–180, 1987.

Baab DA, Johnson RH. The effect of a new electric toothbrush on supragingival plaque and gingivitis. J Periodontol 60:336–341, 1989.

Baderstein A, Nilveus R, Egelberg J. Effect of nonsurgical therapy. II. Severely advanced periodontitis. J Clin Periodontol 11:63–76, 1984a.

Baderstein A, Nilveus R, Egelberg J. Effect of nonsurgical therapy. III. Single versus repeated instrumentation. J Clin Periodontol 11:114–124, 1984b.

Baer PN, Everett FG. Periodontosis—A problem in orthodontics. J Periodontol 46:559–561, 1975.

Balanyk TE. Sanguinarine: Comparisons of antiplaque/antigingivitis reports. Clin Prev Dent 12: 18–25, 1990.

Balenseifen JW, Madonia JV. Study of dental plaque in orthodontic patients. J Dent Res 49: 320–324, 1970.

Barbakow F, Lutz F, Imfeld T. A review of methods to determine the relative abrasion of dentifrices and prophylaxis pastes. Quintessence Int 18:23–28, 1987a.

Barbakow F, Lutz F, Imfeld T. Relative dentin abrasion by dentifrices and prophylaxis pastes. Implications for clinicians, manufacturers, and patients. Quintessence Int 18:29–34, 1987b.

Barkmeier WW, Shaffer SE, Gwinnet AJ. Effects of 15 vs 60 seconds enamel acid conditioning on adhesion and morphology. Oper Dent 11: 111–116, 1986.

Barnes CM, Russell CM, Gerbo LR, Wells BR, Barnes DW. Effects of an air-powder polishing system on orthodontically bracketed and banded teeth. Am J Orthod Dentofac Orthop 97:74–81, 1990.

Bergendal T, Forsgren L, Kvint S, Löwstedt E. The effect of an air-abrasive instrument on soft and hard tissue around osseointegrated implants. Swed Dent J 14:219–223, 1990.

Bergenholtz A, Brithon J. Plaque removal by dental floss or toothpicks. An intra-individual comparative study. J Clin Periodontol 7: 516–524, 1980.

Berglund LJ, Small CL. Effective oral hygiene for orthodontic patients. J Clin Orthod 24:315–320, 1990.

Bergman G, Linden LA. The action of the explorer on incipient caries. Svensk Tandlak Tidskr 62:629–634, 1969.

Berman DS, Slack GL. Susceptibility of tooth surfaces to carious attack. A longitudinal study. Br Dent J 148:134–135, 1973.

Bernimoulin JP, Curilovic Z. Gingival recession and tooth mobility. J Clin Periodontol 4: 107–114, 1977.

Bickel M, Geering AH. Zur bakteriellen Besiedlung der Prothesenbasis. Schweiz Monatsschr Zahnheilkd 92:741–745, 1982.

Bille J, Thylstrup A. Radiographic diagnosis and clinical tissue changes in relation to treatment of approximal carious lesions. Caries Res 16:1–6, 1982.

Birkeland JM, Broch L, Jorkjend L. Caries experience as predictor for caries incidence. Community Dent Oral Epidemiol 4:66–69, 1976.

Bishara SE, Andreasen G. Third molars: a review. Am J Orthod 83:131–137, 1983.

Bishara SE, Chan D, Abadir EA. The effect on the bonding strength of orthodontic brackets of fluoride application after etching. Am J Orthod Dentofac Orthop 95:259–260, 1989.

Block PL, Lobene RR, Derdivanis JP. A two-tone dye test for dental plaque. J Periodontol 43: 423–426, 1972.

Bonesvoll P, Gjermo P. A comparison between chlorhexidine and some quarternary ammonium compounds with regard to retention, salivary concentration and plaque-inhibiting effect in the human mouth after mouth rinses. Arch Oral Biol 23:289–294, 1978.

Bonesvoll P, Løkken P, Rølla G, Paus PN. Retention of chlorhexidine in the human oral cavity after mouth rinses. Arch Oral Biol 19: 209–212, 1974.

Boyd RL, Baumrind S. Periodontal considerations on the use of bonds or bands in molars in adolescents and adults. Angle Orthod 62: 117–126, 1992.

Boyd RL, Murray P, Robertson PB. Effect of rotary electric toothbrush versus manual toothbrush on periodontal status during orthodontic treatment. Am J Orthod Dentofac Orthop 96:342–347, 1989.

Boyd RL, Leggott PJ, Quinn RS, Eakle WS, Chambers D. Periodontal implications of orthodontic treatment in adults with reduced or normal periodontal tissues versus those of adolescents. Am J Orthod Dentofac Orthop 96:191–199, 1989.

Brecx M, Netuschil L, Reichert B, Schreil G. Efficacy of Listerine, Meridol and chlorhexidine mouthrinses on plaque, gingivitis and plaque bacteria vitality. J Clin Periodontol 17:292–297, 1990.

Brooks JD, Merzt-Fairhurst EJ, Della-Giustina VE, Williams JE, Fairhurst CW. A comparative study of two pit and fissure sealants—two year results. J Am Dent Assoc 98:722–725, 1979.

Brown FH, Ogletree RC, Houston GD. Pneumoparotitis associated with the use of an air-powder prophylaxis unit. J Periodontol 63: 642–644, 1992.

Brown LJ. Periodontal status in the United States, 1988–91: prevalence, extent, and demographic variation. J Dent Res (special issue) 75:672–683, 1996.

Brunelle JA, Bhat M, Lipton JA. Prevalence and distribution of selected occlusal characteristics in the US population, 1988–1991. J Dent Res 75 (spec no):706–713, 1996.

Brunelle JA, Miller AJ, Smith JI. DMFS in US children with and without lifelong exposure to water fluoridation. J Dent Res 62 (special issue):203, abstract 302, 1983.

Buckley LA. The relationship between malocclusion, gingival inflammation, plaque and calculus. J Periodontol 52:35–40, 1981.

Burt BA. The changing patterns of systemic fluoride intake. J Dent Res 71:1228–1237, 1992.

Caufield PW, Gibbons RJ. Suppression of Streptococcus mutans in mouths of humans by a dental prophylaxis and topically-applied iodine. J Dent Res 58:1317–1326, 1979.

Ceen RF, Gwinnett AJ. White spot formation associated with sealants used in orthodontics. Pediatr Dent 3:174–178, 1981.

Chaet R, Wei SHY. The effect of fluoride impregnated dental floss on enamel fluoride uptake in vitro and *Streptococcus mutans* colonization in vivo. J Dent Child 2:122–126, 1977.

Chatterjee R, Kleinberg I. Effect of orthodontic band placement on the chemical composition of human incisor tooth plaque. Arch Oral Biol 24: 97–100, 1979.

Ciancio SG, Mather ML, Zambon JJ, Reynolds HS. Effect of chemotherapeutic agent delivered by an oral irrigation device on plaque, gingivitis, and subgingival microflora. J Periodontol 6:310, 1989.

Claffey N. Decision making in periodontal therapy. J Clin Periodontol 18:384–389, 1991.

Clark DC. Trends in prevalence of dental fluorosis in North America. Community Dent Oral Epidemiol 22:148–152, 1994.

Clark DC, Stamm JW, Tessier C. Results of a 32-month fluoride varnish study in Sherbrooke and Lac-Megantic, Canada. J Am Dent Assoc 111: 949–953, 1985.

Clark JR. Oral hygiene in the orthodontic practice. Motivation, responsibilities, and concepts. Am J Orthod 69:72–82, 1976.

Clifford M. Physical attractiveness and academic performance. Child Stud J 5:201–275, 1975.

Clinical Research Associates. Oral prophylaxis, Prophy Jet. Clin Res Assoc 5 (1):1–2, 1981.

Coontz EJ. The effectiveness of a new home plaque-removal instrument on plaque removal. Compend Contin Educ Dent (Suppl 6):117–122, 1985.

Corbett JA, Brown LR, Keene HJ, Horton IM. Comparison of *Streptococcus mutans* concentrations in non-banded and banded orthodontic patients. J Dent Res 60:1936–1942, 1981.

Crossner C-G. Salivary lactobacillus counts in the prediction of caries activity. Community Dent Oral Epidemiol 9:182–190, 1981.

Crossner C-G, Hagberg C. A clinical and microbiological evaluation of the Dentocult dip-slide test. Swed Dent J 1:85–94, 1977.

Crossner C-G, Unell L. Salivary lactobacillus counts as a diagnostic and didactic tool in caries prevention. Community Dent Oral Epidemiol 14: 156–160, 1986.

Cummins D. Zinc citrate/Triclosan: A new antiplaque system for the control of plaque and prevention of gingivitis: Short-term clinical studies and mode of action studies. J Clin Periodontol 18:455–461, 1991.

Curtress TW, Brown RH, Barker DS. Effects on plaque and gingivitis of a chlorhexidine dental gel in the mentally retarded. Community Dent Oral Epidemiol 5:78–83, 1977.

Dahlén G. Role of suspected periodontopathogens in microbiological monitoring of periodontitis. Adv Dent Res 7:163–174, 1993.

Davies TM, Shaw WC, Worthington HV, Addy M, Dummer P, Kingdon A. The effect of orthodontic treatment on plaque and gingivitis. Am J Orthod Dentofac Orthop 99:157–161, 1991.

Dean HT. Endemic fluorosis and its relation to dental caries. Publ Health Rep 53:1443–1452, 1938.

De Bruyn H, Arends J. Fluoride varnishes—A review. J Biol Buccale 15:71–82, 1987.

De Bruyn H, Buskes H. Die kariepräventive Wirkung von Fluor Protector und Duraphat unter stark kariogenen Bedingungen. Oralprophylaxe 1:61–67, 1988.

Declerck HA, Coster WJ, Adriaens PA. Quantification of supragingival plaque formation by automatic image analysis. J Dent Res 68:899, 1989.

Dederich N, Gulevich T, Reid A. The effect of rubber cup vs an air-powder abrasive system on root surfaces. Can Dent Hyg/Probe 23: 135–137, 1989.

De graene GP, Martens C, Dermaut R. The invasive pit- and fissure-sealing technique in pediatric dentistry—an SEM study of a preventive restoration. J Dent Child 55:34–42, 1988.

De Leifde B, Herbison GP. Prevalence of developmental defects of enamel and dental caries in New Zealand children receiving different fluoride supplementation. Community Dent Oral Epidemiol 13: 164–167, 1985.

Dénes J, Lindner Z, Szivós I, Hepp K. Untersuchungen über den Erfolg eines Programms zur Mundhygiene-Motivation bei Patienten mit festsitzenden Apparaturen. Fortschr Kieferorthop 47:212–214, 1986.

DePaola LG, Overholser CD, Meiller TF, Minah GE, Niehaus C. Chemotherapeutic inhibition of supragingival dental plaque and gingivitis development. J Clin Periodontol 16:311–315, 1989.

De yong HP, de Boer P, Busscher HJ, van Pelt AW, Arends J. Surface free energy changes of human enamel during pellicle formation. An in vivo study. Caries Res 18:408–415, 1984.

Diamanti-Kipioti A, Gusberti FA, Lang NP. Clinical and microbiological effects of fixed orthodontic appliances. J Clin Periodontol 14:326–333, 1987.

Diedrich P. Keimbesiedlung und verschiedene Reinigungsverfahren kieferorthopädischer Geräte. Fortschr Kieferorthop 50:231–239, 1989.

Disney JA, Stamm JW, Graves RC, Bohannan HM, Abernathy JR, Zack DD. The University of North Carolina Caries Risk Assessment study: further developments in caries risk prediction. Community Dent Oral Epidemiol 20:64–75, 1992.

Dowell TB. The use of toothpaste in infancy. Br Dent J 150:247–249, 1981.

Downer MC. Concurrent validity of an epidemiological diagnostic system for caries with the histological appearance of extracted teeth as validating criterion. Caries Res 9:231–246, 1975.

Downer MC. Changing patterns of disease in the Western World. In: Guggenheim B (ed). Cariology Today. Basel, Karger, 1–12, 1984.

Duff EJ. Total and ionic fluoride in milk. Caries Res 15:406–408, 1981.

Dünninger P, Pieper K. Ergebnisse zur Prävalenz von Karies und Dentalfluorose. In: Micheelis W, Bauch J (eds): Mundgesundheitszustand und -verhalten in der Bundesrepublik Deutschland. Cologne, Deutscher Ärzte-Verlag, 205–260, 1991.

Dreizen S, Brown LR. Xerostomia and dental caries. In: Stiles HM, Loesche WJ, O'Brien TC (eds). Microbial Aspects of Dental Caries. Vol I. Washington/London, Information Retrieval Inc, 263–273, 1976.

Dzink JL, Socransky SS. Comparative in vitro activity of sanguinarine against oral microbial isolates. Antimicrob Agents Chemother 27:663–665, 1985.

Eakle WS, Ford C, Boyd R. Depth of penetration in periodontal pockets with oral irrigation. J Clin Periodontol 13:39–44, 1986.

Edgar WM, Geddes DA. Chewing gum and dental health—A review. Br Dent J 168:173–177, 1990.

Ehmer U. Motivation zur kieferorthopädischen Behandlung aus der Sicht des Patienten und seiner Eltern in Beziehung zu objektiven Symptomen der Dysgnathie. Fortschr Kieferorthop 42:441–450, 1981.

Eisenberg AD, Young DA, Fan J. Antimicrobial activity of sanguinarine and zinc. J Dent Res 64 (special issue): abstract 341, 1985.

Ekstrand J, Koch G. Systemic fluoride absorption following fluoride gel application. J Dent Res 59:1067, 1980.

Ekstrand J, Koch G, Petersson LG. Plasma fluoride concentration and urinary fluoride excretion in children following application of the fluoride-containing varnish Duraphat. Caries Res 14:185–189, 1980.

Ekstrand K, Qvist V, Thyltrup A. Light microscope study of the effect of probing in occlusal surfaces. Caries Res 21:368–374, 1987.

Eliades GC, Tzoutzas JG, Vougiouklakis GJ. Surface alterations on dental restorative materials subjected to an air-powder abrasive instrument. J Prosthet Dent 65:27–33, 1991.

Eliasson LA, Hugoson A, Kürol J, Siwe H. The effects of orthodontic treatment on periodontal tissues in patients with reduced periodontal support. Eur J Orthod 4:1–9, 1982.

El-Nadeef MAI, Bratthall D. Intraindividual variations in counts of mutans streptococci measured by "Strip mutans" method. Scand J Dent Res 99:8–12, 1991.

Emilson CG. Effect of chlorhexidine gel treatment on Streptococcus mutans population in human saliva and dental plaque. Scand J Dent Res 89:239–246, 1981.

Emilson CG, Axelsson P, Kallenberg L. Effect of mechanical and chemical plaque control measures on oral microflora in schoolchildren. Community Dent Oral Epidemiol 10:111–116, 1982.

Emilson CG. Potential efficacy of chlorhexidine against mutans streptococci and human dental caries. J Dent Res 73:682–91, 1994.

Ericsson I, Thilander B, Lindhe J, Okamoto H. The effect of orthodontic tilting movements on the periodontal tissues of infected and non-infected dentitions in dogs. J Clin Periodontol 4:278–293, 1977.

Fadel B, Jost-Brinkmann P-G, Miethke R-R. Verfärbung von Alastiks und elastichen Ketten unter dem Einfluss verschiedener Nahrungs-und Genussmittel. Prakt Kieferorthop 6:279–286, 1992.

Fédération Dentaire Internationale/World Health Organization. Changing patterns of oral health and implications for oral health manpower. Part I. Int Dent J 35:235–251, 1985.

Fejerskov O. Strategies in the design of preventive programs. Adv Dent Res 9:82–88, 1995.

Fejerskov O, Manji F, Baelum V. The nature and mechanisms of dental fluorosis in man. J Dent Res 69 (special issue):692–700, 1990.

Feliu JL. Long term benefits of orthodontic treatment on oral hygiene. Am J Orthod 82:473–477, 1982.

Finkelstein P, Yost KG, Grossman E. Mechanical devices versus antimicrobial rinses in plaque and gingivitis reduction. Clin Prev Dent 12:8–11, 1990.

Finster W, Riethe P. Experimentelle und bakteriologische Untersuchungen an Kupferzementen. Zahnärztl Welt 64:340–344, 1963.

Flemming TF, Newman MG, Doherty FM, Grossman E, Meckle AH, Bakdash B. Supragingival irrigation with 0.06% chlorhexidine in naturally occurring gingivitis. I. 6 month clinical observations. J Periodontol 61:112–117, 1990.

Flores de Jacoby L, Müller HP. Zusammensetzung der subgingivalen Mundflora bei Trägern abnehmbarer kieferorthopädischer Geräte. Dtsch Zahnärztl Z 37:925–928, 1982.

Food and Agriculture Organization/World Health Organization. Expert committee on food additives. FAO Nutrition Meetings, Report Series 55, 1975.

Forss H, Seppä L. Prevention of enamel demineralization adjacent to glass ionomer filling material. Scand J Dent Res 98:173–178, 1990.

Forsten L. Short- and long-term fluoride release from glass ionomers and other fluoride-containing filling material in vitro. Scand J Dent Res 98:179–185, 1990.

Fox CH. New considerations in the prevalence of periodontal disease. Curr Opin Dent 2:5-11, 1992.

Frandsen A. Mechanical oral hygiene practices. State-of-the-science review. In: Löe H, Kleinman DV (eds): Dental Plaque Control Measures and Oral Hygiene Practices. Oxford, IRL Press: 93–116, 1986.

Freundorfer A, Purucker P, Miethke R-R. Kieferorthopädische Behandlungen können ohne professionelle Mundhygiene zu dauerhaften Veränderungen der subgingivalen Plaqueflora führen. Prakt Kieferorthop 7:187–200, 1993.

Friedman M, Harari D, Rax H, Golomb G, Brayer L. Plaque inhibition by sustained release of chlorhexidine from removable appliances. J Dent Res 64:1319–1321, 1985.

Fure S, Emilson CG. Effect of chlorhexidine gel treatment supplemented with chlorhexidine varnish and resin on mutans streptococci and Actinomyces on root surfaces. Caries Res 24:242–247, 1990.

Galil KA, Gwinnett AJ. Human tooth-fissure contents and their progressive mineralization. Arch Oral Biol 20:559–563, 1975.

Geiger AM, Gorelick L, Gwinnett AJ, Griswold PG. The effect of a fluoride program on white spot formation during orthodontic treatment. Am J Orthod Dentofac Orthop 93:29–37, 1988.

Geiger AM, Wasserman BH, Turgeon LR. Relation of occlusion and periodontal disease. Part VIII. Relationship of crowding and spacing to periodontal destruction and gingival inflammation. J Periodontol 45:43–49, 1974.

Genco RJ. Pharmaceuticals and periodontal diseases. J Am Dent Assoc 125 (suppl):11S–19S, 1994.

Genco RJ. Current view of risk factors for periodontal diseases. J Periodontol 67:1041–1049, 1996.

Ghafari J. Problems associated with ceramic brackets suggest limiting use to selected teeth. Angle Orthod 62:145–152, 1992.

Ghafari J, Locke SA, Bentley JM. Longitudinal evaluation of the treatment priority index TPI. Am J Orthod Dentofac Orthop 96:382–389, 1989.

Gjermo P. Contemporary use of agents in the control of progressive periodontitis. Int Dent J 43:499–505, 1993.

Glass RL. The first international conference on the declining prevalence of dental caries. J Dent Res 61:1301–1383, 1982.

Going RE, Loesche WJ, Grainger DA, Syed SA. The viability of microorganisms in carious lesions five years after covering with a fissure sealant. J Am Dent Assoc 97:455–462, 1978.

Goodson JM. Pharmacokinetic principles controlling efficacy of oral therapy. J Dent Res 68:1625–1632, 1989.

Gordon JM, Frascella JA, Reardon RC. A clinical study of the safety and efficacy of a novel electric interdental cleaning device. J Clin Dent 7:70–73, 1996.

Gorelick L, Geiger AM, Gwinnet AJ. Incidence of white spot formation after banding and bonding. Am J Orthod 81:93–98, 1982.

Gorfil C, Nordenberg D, Liberman R, Ben-Amar A. The effect of ultrasonic cleaning and air polishing on the marginal integrity of radicular amalgam and composite resin restorations. An in vitro study. J Clin Periodontol 16:137–139, 1989.

Gorman JC, Hilgers JJ, Smith JR. Lingual orthodontics. A status report. Part 4. Diagnosis and treatment planning. J Clin Orthod 17:26–35, 1983.

Greenstein G. Diagnosis of periodontal diseases. Compend Contin Educ Dent 15:750–772, 1994.

Gröndahl H-G. Radiographic caries diagnosis and treatment decisions. Swed Dent J 3:109–117, 1979.

Grossman E. Effectiveness of a pre-brushing mouthrinse under single-trial and home-use conditions. Clin Prev Dent 10:3–6, 1988.

Gwinnett JA, Ceen F. Plaque distribution on bonded brackets. Am J Orthod 75:667–677, 1979.

Haffajee AD, Socransky SS, Goodson JM. Clinical predictors of destructive periodontal disease activities. J Clin Periodontol 10:257–265, 1983.

Haffajee AD, Socransky SS, Lindhe J, Kent RL, Okamoto H, Yoneyama T. Clinical risk indicators for periodontal attachment loss. J Clin Periodontol 18:117–125, 1991.

Handelman SL, Leverett DH, Iker HP. Longitudinal radiographic evaluation of the progress of caries under sealants. J Pedod 9: 119–126, 1985.

Hannah JJ, Johnson JD, Kuftinec MM. Long-term clinical evaluation of toothpaste and oral rinse containing sanguinaria extract in controlling plaque, gingival inflammation, and sulcular bleeding during orthodontic treatment. Am J Orthod Dentofac Orthop 96:199–207, 1989.

Hannemann M, Diedrich P. Der Einsatz des Prophy-Jet-Gerätes zur Schmelzpolitur nach der Bracketentfernung. Fortschr Kieferorthop 47: 317–326, 1986.

Harper DS, Mueller LJ, Fine JB, Gordon J, Laster LL. Clinical efficacy of a dentifrice and oral rinse containing sanguinaria extract and zinc chloride during 6 months of use. J Periodontol 61:352–358, 1990.

Hartmann F, Jeromin R, Flores de Jacoby L. Untersuchungen über den parodontalen Zustand jugendlicher Träger festsitzender kieferorthopädischer Geräte. Dtsch Zahnärztl Z 37:585–589, 1982.

Hastreiter RJ. Is 0.4% stannous fluoride gel an effective agent for the prevention of oral diseases? J Am Dent Assoc 118:205–208, 1989.

Hattab FN, Wei SHY. Dietary sources of fluoride for infants and children in Hong Kong. Pediatr Dent 10:13–18, 1988.

Heikinheimo K. Need of orthodontic treatment and prevalence of craniomandibular dysfunction in Finnish children. Proc Finn Dent Soc 86: 38–138, 1990.

Heintze SD. Screening von Individuen mit hohem Kariesrisikom—Evaluation verschiedener Karies-prädiktoren im multifaktoriellen Modell [thesis]. Free University, Berlin, 1991.

Heintze SD. Versiegelung von Fissuren und Grübchen—Indikationen, Techniken und Alternativen I. ZWR 105:46–50, 1996a.

Heintze SD. Versiegelung von Fissuren und Grübchen—Indikationen, Techniken und Alternativen II. ZWR 105:128–131, 1996b.

Heintze SD, Bastos JRM, Roversi MJ. The prevalence of dental caries and fluorosis in 6- to 44-year-olds in two Brazilian cities with and without water fluoridation. Sixth World Congress on Preventive Dentistry, Cape Town, South Africa, 1997.

Heintze SD, Busse H, Roulet J-F. Evaluation of different caries predictors in a multifactorial model. In: Morioka T (ed): Proceedings of the 3rd World Congress on Preventive Dentistry, Fukuoka, Japan, 213–215, 1991.

Heintze SD, Jost-Brinkmann P-G, Loundos J. Effectiveness of three different types of electrical toothbrushes compared with a manual technique in orthodontic patients. Am J Orthod Dentofac Orthop 110:630–638, 1996.

Heintze SD, Roulet J-F. Inter-examiner variability in estimating lactobacilli dip-slides. J Dent Res 71:abstract 189, 1992.

Helm S, Kreiborg S, Solow B. Psychological implications of malocclusions: A 15-year follow-up study in 30 year old Danes. Am J Orthod 87:110–118, 1985.

Helm S, Petersen PE. Causal relation between malocclusion and caries. Acta Odontol Scand 47:217–221, 1989a.

Helm S, Petersen PE. Causal relation between malocclusion and periodontal health. Acta Odontol Scand 47:223–228, 1989b.

Herzberg MC, Meyer MW. Effects of oral flora on platelets: possible consequences in cardiovascular disease. J Periodontol 67:1138–1142, 1996.

Hickel R. Indikation und Materialien für die Fissurenversiegelung. Zahnärztl Welt 98:944–951, 1989.

Hildebrandt GH, Pape JHR, Syed SA, Gregory WA, Friedman M. Effect of slow-release chlorhexidine mouthguards on the levels of selected salivary bacteria. Caries Res 26:268–274, 1992.

Hiller ME, Rankine CA, Majo JA. The anticariogenic potential of fluoride-releasing resin. J La Dent Assoc 49:7–8, 1990.

Holm G-B, Holst K, Mejàre I. The caries preventive effect of a fluoride varnish in the fissures of first permanent molars. Acta Odontol Scand 42:193–197, 1984.

Honkala E, Nyyssönen V, Kolmakow S, Lammi S. Factors predicting caries risk in children. Scand J Dent Res 92:134–140, 1984.

Horowitz AM, Suomi JD, Peterson JK, Lyman BA. Effect of supervised daily plaque removal by children: Results after third and final year. J Dent Res 56 (special issue): abstract 170, 1977.

Horowitz HS. Misuse of topically applied fluorides. J Am Soc Prev Dent 7:15–16, 1977.

Hosoya Y, Johnston JW. Evaluation of various cleaning and polishing methods on primary enamel. J Pedod 13:253–269, 1989.

Hotz PR. Prävention von Karies und Gingivitis bei der kieferorthopädischen Behandlung. Schweiz Monatsschr Zahnheilkd 92:880–888, 1982.

Hotz PR, Dula KF, Blaser M. Der Einfluss verschiedener Zahnbürsten und Zahnreinigungstechniken auf die interdentale Belagsentfernung bei Zähnen ohne und mit festsitzenden kieferorthopädischen Apparaturen. Ein Versuch am Modell. Schweiz Monatsschr Zahnheilkd 94:572–579, 1984.

Houpt M, Sheykholeslam Z. The clinical effectiveness of Delton fissure sealant after one year. J Dent Child 45:130–132, 1978.

Huber SJ, Vernino AR, Nanda RS. Professional prophylaxis and its effect on the periodontium of full-banded orthodontic patients. Am J Orthod Dentofac Orthop 91:321–327, 1987.

Hugoson A, Koch G, Bergendal T, Laurell L, Lundren D. Caries prevalence and distribution in individuals aged 20-80 years in Jönköping, Sweden, 1973 and 1983. Swed Dent J 12:133–140, 1988.

Huizinga ED. Antimicrobial varnish and root surface caries. (PhD thesis.) University of Groningen, 1991.

Huizinga ED, Arends J. The effect of an antimicrobial-containing varnish on enamel caries in situ. A comparison between the in situ efficacy of the varnish on caries in enamel and root surface. Caries Res 24:130–132, 1990.

Huizinga ED, Ruben J, Arends J. Effect of an antimicrobial-containing varnish on root demineralisation in situ. Caries Res 24:130–132, 1990.

Huizinga ED, Ruben J, Arends J. Chlorhexidine and thymol release from a varnish system. J Biol Buccale 19:343–348, 1991.

Huser MC, Baehni PC, Lang R. Effects of orthodontic bands on microbiological and clinical parameters. Am J Orthod Dentofac Orthop 97:213–218, 1990.

Imfeld T, Saxer UP. Stellungnahme zum Mundspülmittel Plax. Schweiz Monatsschr Zahnheilkd 100:893, 1990.

Ingervall B. The influence of orthodontic appliances on caries frequency. Odontol Rev 13: 175–190, 1962.

Ingervall B, Jacobsson U, Nyman S. A clinical study of the relationhip between crowding of teeth, plaque and gingival condition. J Clin Periodontol 4:214–222, 1977.

Jarvinen S. Traumatic injuries to upper permanent incisors related to age and upper incisal overjet. Acta Odontol Scand 37:335–338, 1979.

Jeffcoat MK, Jeffcoat RL, Jens SC, Captain K. A new periodontal probe with automated cemento-enamel junction detection. J Clin Periodontol 13:276–280, 1986.

Jeffcoat MK, McGuire M, Newman MG. Evidence-based periodontal treatment. J Am Dent Assoc 128:713–724, 1997.

Jeffcoat MK, Reddy MS. Progression of probing attachment loss in adult periodontitis. J Periodontol 62:185–189, 1991.

Jensen B, Bratthall D. A new method for the estimation of mutans streptococci in human saliva. J Dent Res 68:468–471, 1989.

Jensen ØE, Billings RJ, Featherstone DB. Clinical evaluation of Fluoroshield and fissure sealant. Clin Prev Dent 12:24–27, 1990.

Johnsen DC, Pappas LR, Cannon D, Goodman SJ. Social factors and diet diaries of caries-free and high-caries 2- to 7-year olds presenting for dental care in West Virginia. Pediatr Dent 2:279–286, 1980.

Jost-Brinkmann P-G. The influence of air polishers on tooth enamel: in-vitro study. J Orofac Orthop 59:1–16, 1998.

Jost-Brinkmann P-G, Dürr W, Miethke R-R. Thermodebonding von Metall- und Keramikbrackets. Prakt Kieferorthop 3:249–256, 1989.

Jost-Brinkmann P-G, Heintze SD, Loundos J. Studie zur Wirksamkeit elektrischer Zahnbürsten bei Multiband-Patienten. Kieferorthop 8:235–246, 1994.

Jost-Brinkmann P-G, Miethke R-R. Indirektes Kleben. Ein klinischer Bericht. Schweiz Monatsschr Zahnheilkd 98:1356–1363, 1988.

Jost-Brinkmann P-G, Nündel M, Riedel E, Schrinner H-U, Miethke R-R. Adsorption und Permeation von Aminosäuren durch einen kupferhaltigen und einen kupferfreien Zinkphosphatzement sowie Demineralisation von Zahnschmelz unter Zementspalten. ZWR 103: 158–162, 1994.

Jost-Brinkmann P-G, Rabe H, Miethke R-R. Werkstoffeigenschaften von Zinkphosphatzementen nach verzögertem Abbinden auf gekühlten Platten. Fortschr Kieferorthop 50:1–11, 1989.

Jost-Brinkmann P-G, Stein H, Miethke R-R, Nakata M. Histologic investigation of the human pulp after thermodebonding of metal and ceramic brackets. Am J Orthod Dentofac Orthop 102:410–417, 1992.

Kaste LM, Selwitz RH, Oldakowski RJ, Brunelle JA, Winn DM, Brown LJ. Coronal caries in the primary and permanent dentition of children and adolescents 1–17 years of age: United States, 1988–1991. J Dent Res 75 (special issue): 631–641, 1996.

Katz RV. An epidemiological study of the relationship between various states of occlusion and the pathological conditions of dental caries and periodontal disease. J Dent Res 56:433–439, 1977.

Kaufman AY, Tal H, Perlmutter S, Shwartz MM. Reduction of dental plaque formation by chlorhexidine dihydrochloride lozenges. J Periodont Res 24:59–62, 1989.

Kess K, Koch R, Witt E. Ergebnisse zur Prävalenz von Zahnfehlstellungen bzw. Okklusionsstörungen. In: Micheelis W, Bauch J (eds): Mundgesundheitszustand und—verhalten in der Bundesrepublik Deutschland. Cologne, Deutscher Ärzte-Verlag, 297–334, 1991.

Kieser JB, Wade AB. Use of food colourants as plaque disclosing agents. J Clin Periodontol 3:200–207, 1976.

Killoy WJ, Love JW, Love J, Fedi PJ, Tira DE. The effectiveness of a counter-rotary action powered toothbrush and conventional toothbrush on plaque removal and gingival bleeding. A short term study. J Periodontol 60:473-477, 1989.

Kingman A, Little W, Gomes I, Heifetz SB, Driscoll WS, Sheats R, Supan P. Salivary levels of Streptococcus mutans and lactobacilli and dental caries experiences in a US adolescent population. Community Dent Oral Epidemiol 16: 98–103, 1988.

Kipioti A, Tsamis A, Mitsis F. Disclosing agents in plaque control. Evaluation of their role during periodontal treatment. Clin Prev Dent 6:9–13, 1984.

Kirkegaard E, Petersen G, Poulsen S. Caries preventive effect of Duraphat varnish applications versus fluoride mouthrinses. Caries Res 20: 548–555, 1986.

Klock B, Emilson C, Lin S, Gustavsdotte M, Olhede-Westerlun AM. Prediction of caries activity in children with today's low caries incidence. Community Dent Oral Epidemiol 17:285–288, 1989.

Klock B, Krasse B. A comparison between different methods for prediction of caries activity. Scand J Dent Res 87:129–139, 1979.

Klock B, Serling J, Kinder S, Manwell MA, Tinanoff N. Comparison of effect of SnF_2 and NaF mouthrinses on caries incidence, salivary S mutans and gingivitis in high caries prevalent adults. Scand J Dent Res 93:213–217, 1985.

Koch G, Hagberg M, Petersson LG. Fluoride uptake on dry versus water-saliva wetted human enamel surfaces in vitro after topical application of a varnish (Duraphat) containing fluoride. Swed Dent J 12:221–225, 1988.

Koch G, Petersson LG, Ryden H. Effect of a fluoride varnish treatment every six months compared with weekly mouthrinses with 0.2 percent NaF solutions on dental caries. Swed Dent J 3: 39–55, 1979.

Köhler B, Andréen I, Jonsson B. The effect of caries-preventive measures in mothers on dental caries and the oral presence of the bacteria Streptococcus mutans and lactobacilli in their children. Arch Oral Biol 29:879–883, 1984.

Köhler B, Bratthall D. Intrafamilial levels of Streptococcus mutans and some aspects of the bacterial transmission. Scand J Dent Res 86: 35–42, 1978.

Köhler B, Bratthall D. Practical method to facilitate estimation of Streptococcus mutans levels in saliva. J Clin Microbiol 95:584–588, 1979.

Köhler B, Bratthall D, Krasse B. Preventive measures in mothers influence the establishment of the bacterium Streptococcus mutans in their infants. Arch Oral Biol 28:225–231, 1983.

Kokich VG, Mathews DP. Managing and coordinating treatment of periodontal problems. PSCO Bull 61:37–41, 1989.

Konturri-Närhi V, Markkanen S, Markkanen H. Effects of airpolishing on dental plaque removal and hard tissues as evaluated by scanning electron microscopy. J Periodontol 61:334–338, 1990.

Krasse B. Die Quintessenz des Kariesrisikos. Beurteilung—Behandlung—Kontrolle. Berlin, Quintessenz, 1986.

Krasse B. Biological factors as indicators of future caries. Int Dent J 38:219–225, 1988.

Kremers L, Unterer S, Lampert F. Mundhygiene für Träger festsitzender kieferorthopädischer Apparaturen. Fortschr Kieferorthop 44:147–152, 1983.

Kristoffersson K, Axelsson P, Bratthall D. Effect of a professional tooth cleaning program on interdentally localized Streptococcus mutans. Caries Res 18:385–390, 1984.

Kristoffersson K, Gröndahl H-G, Bratthall D. The more Streptococcus mutans, the more caries on approximal surfaces. J Dent Res 64:58–61, 1985.

Kweider M, Lowe GD, Murray GD, Kinane DF, McGowan DA. Dental disease, fibrinogen and white cell count; links with myocardial infarction? Scott Med J 38:73–74, 1993.

Lamster IB. Evaluation of components of gingival crevicular fluid as diagnostic tests. Ann Periodontol 2:123–137, 1997.

Lamster IB, Celenti RS, Jans NH, Fine JB, Grbic JT. Current status of tests for periodontal disease. Adv Dent Res 7:182–190, 1993.

Lang NP. Chemische Plaquekontrolle. In: Peters S (ed): Prophylaxe. Ein Leitfaden für die zahnärztliche Praxis. Berlin, Quintessenz, 245–267, 1978.

Lang NP, Adler R, Joss A, Nyman S. Absence of bleeding on probing. An indicator of periodontal stability. J Clin Periodontol 17:714–721, 1990.

Lang NP, Brägger U. Periodontal diagnosis in the 1990s. J Clin Periodontol 18:370–379, 1991.

Lang NP, Brecx MC. Chlorhexidine digluconate. An agent for chemical plaque control and prevention of gingival inflammation. J Periodont Res 21 (suppl 16):74–89, 1986.

Lang NP, Corbet EF. Periodontal diagnosis in daily practice. Int Dent J 45:3–15, 1995.

Lang NP, Cumming BR, Löe H. Toothbrushing frequency as it relates to plaque development and gingival health. J Periodontol 44:396–405, 1973.

Lang NP, Hotz P, Graf H, Geering AH, Saxer UP. Longitudinal effects of supervised chlorhexidine mouthrinses in children. J Periodont Res 17: 101–111, 1982.

Lang NP, Räber K. Use of oral irrigators as vehicle for the application of antimicrobial agents in chemical plaque control. J Clin Periodontol 8:177–188, 1981.

Larmas M. A new dip-slide method for the counting of salivary lactobacilli. Proc Finn Dent Soc 71:31–35, 1975.

Le Bell Y, Forsten L. Sealing of preventively enlarged fissures. Acta Odontol Scand 38: 101–104, 1980.

LeCompte EJ, Doyle TE. Oral fluoride retention following various topical application techniques in children. J Dent Res 61:469–472, 1982.

Legott PJ, Boyd RL, Quinn RS, Eakle WS, Chambers DW. Gingival disease pattern during fixed orthodontic treatment adolescents vs adults. J Dent Res 63:309, abstract 1245, 1984.

Lervik T, Haugejorden O. Orthodontic treatment, dental health, and oral health behavior in young Norwegian adults. Angle Orthod 58:381–386, 1988.

Leverett DH, Proskin HM, Featherstone JD, Adair SM, Eisenberg AD, Mundorff SS, Shields CP, Shaffer CL, Billings RJ. Caries risk assessment in a longitudinal discrimination study. J Dent Res 72:538–543, 1993.

Levine RA. A patient-centered periodontal program for the 1990s, Part I. Compend Contin Educ Dent 11:222–231, 1990.

Lindquist B, Edward E, Torell P, Krasse B. Effect of different caries preventive measures in children highly infected with mutans streptococci. Scand J Dent Res 97:330–337, 1988.

Listgarten MA. A perspective on periodontal diagnosis. J Clin Periodontol 13:175–181, 1986.

Lobene RR, Soparkar PM, Newman MB. Long-term evaluation of a prebrushing dental rinse for the control of dental plaque and gingivitis. Clin Prev Dent 12:26–30, 1990.

Löe H, Brown LJ. Early onset periodontitis in the United States of America. J Periodontol 62: 608–616, 1991.

Löe H, von der Fehr F, Schiött CR. Inhibition of experimental caries by plaque prevention. The effect of chlorhexidine mouth rinses. Scand J Dent Res 80:1–9, 1972.

Löe H, Morrison E. Periodontal health and disease in young people: screening for priority care. Int Dent J 36:162–167, 1986.

Loesche WJ. Personal communication, 1990.

Long DE, Killoy WJ. Evaluation of the effectiveness of the Interplak home plaque removal instrument on plaque removal and orthodontic patients. Compend Contin Educ Dent (Suppl 6):156–160, 1985.

Loundos J. Evaluation der Randdichtigkeit zweier ungefüllter, eingefärbter Versieglermaterialien in vitro. Vergleich dreier Prüfmethoden (thesis). Free University, Berlin, 1997.

Lundqvist C. Oral sugar clearance. Odontol Rev 3 (suppl 1):1–37, 1952.

Lundström F, Hamp S-E, Nyman S. Systematic plaque control in children undergoing long-term orthodontic treatment. Eur J Orthod 2:27–39, 1980.

Lundström F, Krasse B. Streptococcus mutans and lactobacilli frequency in orthodontic patients: the effect of chlorhexidine treatments. Eur J Orthod 9:109–116, 1987.

Lutz F, Sener B, Imfeld T, Barbakow F. Self-adjusting abrasiveness: A new technology for prophylaxis pastes. Quintessence Int 24:53–63, 1993a.

Lutz F, Sener B, Imfeld T, Barbakow F, Schüpbach P. Comparison of the efficacy of prophylaxis pastes with conventional abrasives or a new self-adjusting abrasive. Quintessence Int 24: 193–201, 1993b.

Lynch E, Beighton D. A comparison of primary root caries lesions classified according to colour. Caries Res 28:233–239, 1994.

Maijer R, Smith DC. A comparison between zinc phosphate and glass ionomer cement in orthodontics. Am J Orthod Dentofac Orthop 93: 273–279, 1988.

Mäkinen KK. A dietary procedure for preventing dental caries in young adults. J Am Coll Health 41:172-180, 1993.

Mandel ID. Chemotherapeutic agents for controlling plaque and gingivitis. J Clin Periodontol 15: 488–498, 1988.

Manning RH, Edgar WM. Salivary stimulation by chewing gum and its role in the remineralization of caries-like lesions in human enamel in situ. J Clin Dent 3:71-74, 1992.

Marthaler TM. Selektive Intensivprophylaxe zur weitgehenden Verhütung von Zahnkaries, Gingivitis und Parodontitis beim Schulkind. Schweiz Monatsschr Zahnheilk 12:1227–1240, 1975.

Marthaler TM. Clinical cariostatic effects of various fluoride methods and programs. In: Ekstrand J, Fejerskov O, Silverstone LM (eds): Fluoride in Dentistry. Copenhagen, Munksgaard, 252–275, 1988.

Marthaler TM, Mejia R, Toth K, Vines JJ. Caries-preventive salt fluoridation. Caries Res 12 (suppl 1):15–21, 1978.

Martinsson T. Socio-economic investigation of children with high and low caries frequency. III. A dietary study based on information given by the children. Odontol Rev 23:93–114, 1972.

Mattingly JA, Sauer GJ, Yancey JM, Arnold RR. Enhancement of Streptococcus mutans colonization by direct bonded orthodontic appliances. J Dent Res 62:1209–1211, 1983.

McCann JT, Keller DL, La Bounty GL. Remaining dentin/cementum thickness after hand or ultrasonic instrumentation. J Endod 16: 109–113, 1990.

McCourt JW, Cooley RL, Barnwell S. Bond strength of light-cure fluoride-releasing base-liners as orthodontic bracket adhesives. Am J Orthod Dentofac Orthop 100:47–52, 1991.

McLean JW, Wilson AD. Fissure sealing and filling with an adhesive glass-ionomer cement. Br Dent J 136:269–276, 1974.

Mejàre I, Källestal C, Stenlund H, Johansson H. Caries development from 11 to 22 years of age: A prospective radiographic study. Caries Res 32: 10–16, 1998.

Mejàre I, Mjör IA. Glass ionomer and resin-based fissure sealants: A clinical study. Scand J Dent Res 98:345–350, 1990.

Mellberg JR. Evaluation of topical fluoride preparations. J Dent Res 69:771–779, 1990.

Melsen B, Agerbæk N, Eriksen J, Terp S. New attachment through periodontal treatment and orthodontic intrusion. Am J Orthod Dentofac Orthop 94:104–116, 1988.

Mertz-Fairhurst EJ, Schuster GS, Fairhurst CW. Arresting caries by sealants: results of a clinical study. J Am Dent Assoc 112:194–197, 1986.

Miethke R-R, Bernimoulin J-P. Auswirkungen von Bändern und Brackets auf das marginale Parodontium. Fortschr Kieferorthop 49:160–169, 1988.

Miethke R-R, Melsen B. Adult orthodontics and periodontal diseases—A 9-year review of the literature from 1984 to 1993. Prakt Kieferorthop 7:249–262, 1993.

Miethke R-R, Newesely H. Zur Karieprophylaxe bei der kieferorthopädischen Therapie. Kieferorthopädische Kunststoffe mit Fluoridspeicherfunktion. Fortschr Kieferorthop 48:161–166, 1987.

Miethke R-R, Newesely H. Continuous fluoride release from removable appliances. J Clin Orthod 22:490–491, 1988.

Miller J, Hobson P. The relationship between malocclusion, oral cleanliness, gingival conditions and dental caries in school children. Br Dent J 111:43–52, 1961.

Miller RA, McIver JE, Gunsolley JC. Effects of sanguinaria extract on plaque retention and gingival health. J Clin Orthod 22:304–307, 1988.

Mintz SW. Sweetness and power. The place of sugar in modern history. Viking Penguin, New York, 1985.

Mishkin DJ, Engler WO, Javed T, Darby TD, Cobb RL, Coffman MA. A clinical comparison of the effect on the gingiva of the Prophy-Jet and the rubber cup and paste techniques. J Periodontol 57:151-154, 1986.

Mitropoulos CM. A comparison of fibre-optic transillumination with bitewing radiographs. Br Dent J 159:21–23, 1985.

Mixson JM, Eick JD, Tira DE, Moore DL. The effects of variable washing times and techniques on enamel-composite resin bond strength. Quintessence Int 19:179–285, 1988.

Miyazaki H, Pilot T, Leclercq M-H, Barmes DE. Profiles of periodontal conditions in adolescents measured by CPITN. Int Dent J 41:67–73, 1991.

Miyazaki H, Pilot T, Leclercq M-H, Barmes DE. Profiles of periodontal conditions in adults measured by CPITN. Int Dent J 41:74–80, 1991.

Mizrahi E. Enamel demineralization following orthodontic treatment. Am J Orthod 82:62–67, 1982.

Mohlin B, Thilander B. The importance of the relationship between malocclusion and mandibular dysfunction and some clinical applications in adults. Eur J Orthod 6:192–204, 1984.

Munley M, Everett M, Krupa C, Somerman M, Suzuki J. Removal of extrinsic stain by air powder polishing. J Dent Res 69:abstract 356, 1987.

Murray JJ. Efficacy of preventive agents for dental caries. Systemic fluorides: water fluoridation. Caries Res 28 (suppl 1):2–8, 1993.

Murray PA, Boyd RL, Robertson PB. Effect on periodontal status of rotary electric toothbrushes versus manual toothbrushes during periodontal maintenance. II. Microbiological results. J Periodontol 60:390–395, 1989.

National Institute of Dental Research (NIDR). Oral health of United States children: The national survey of dental caries in U.S. school children. NIH Publication 89-2247, 1989.

National Institutes of Health (NIH). Consensus development conference statement on dental sealants in the prevention of tooth decay. J Am Dent Assoc 108:233–236, 1984.

Naylor MN, Murray JJ. Fluorides and dental caries. In: Murray JJ (ed): The Prevention of Dental Disease. Oxford, England, Oxford University Press, 115–199, 1989.

Newbrun E. Cariology. Chicago, Quintessence, 1989.

Newbrun E. Effectiveness of water fluoridation. J Public Health Dent 49:279–289, 1989.

Newbrun E. Current regulations and recommendations concerning water fluoridation, fluoride supplements, and topical fluoride agents. J Dent Res 71:1255–1265, 1992.

Nizel AE. Nutrition in Preventive Dentistry. Science and Practice. Philadelphia, Saunders, 1981.

Norris DS, McInnes-Ledoux P, Schwaninger B, Weinberg R. Retention of orthodontic bands with new fluoride-releasing cements. Am J Orthod 89:206–211, 1986.

Nyman S, Westfelt E, Sarhed G, Karring T. Role of "diseased" root cementum in healing following treatment of periodontal disease. A clinical study. J Clin Periodontol 15:464–468, 1988.

Offenbacher S, Collins JG, Arnold RR. New clinical diagnostic strategies based on pathogenesis of disease. J Periodontal Res 28:523–535, 1993a.

Offenbacher S, Collins JG, Heasman PA. Diagnostic potential of host response mediators. Adv Dent Res 7:175–181, 1993b.

Øgaard B. Incidence of filled surfaces from 10-18 years of age in an orthodontically treated and untreated group in Norway. Eur J Orthod 11:116–119, 1989.

Øgaard B. Prevalence of white spot lesions in 19-year-olds—a study on untreated and orthodontically treated persons 5 years after treatment. Am J Orthod Dentofac Orthop 96:423–427, 1989.

Øgaard B, Rølla G, Arends J. Orthodontic appliances and enamel demineralization. Part 1. Lesion development. Am J Orthod Dentofac Orthop 94:68–73, 1988a.

Øgaard B, Rølla G, Helgeland K. Fluoride retention in sound and demineralized enamel in vivo after treatment with a fluoride varnish (Duraphat). Scand J Dent Res 92:190–197, 1984.

Øgaard B, Rølla G, Ruben J, Arends J. Microradiographic study of demineralization of shark enamel in a human caries model. Scand J Dent Res 96:209–211, 1988b.

O'Leary TJ, Drake RB, Naylor JE. The plaque control record. J Periodontol 43:38, 1972.

Oliver RG, Howe GS, Scanning electron microscope appearance of the enamel/composite/bracket areas using different methods of surface enamel treatment, composite mix and bracket loading. Br J Orthod 16:39–46, 1989.

O'Mullane D, Clarkson J, Holland T, O'Hickey S, Whelton H. Children's dental health in Ireland. Dublin, Government publications, 1984.

Ong G. The effectiveness of 3 types of dental floss for interdental plaque removal. J Clin Periodontol 17:463–466, 1990.

O'Reilly MM, Featherstone JD. Demineralization and remineralization around orthodontic appliances. An in vivo study. Am J Orthod Dentofac Orthop 92:33–40, 1987.

Ørstavik D. Salivary factors in initial plaque formation. In: Berkeley RCW, Lynch JM, Melling J, Rutter PR, Vincent B (eds): Microbial adhesion to Surfaces. Chichester, Ellis Horwood, 407–423, 1980.

Ørstavik D, Ørstavik J. Two-hour bacterial colonization of dental luting cements in vivo. Acta Odontol Scand 39:115–123, 1981.

Ostela I, Tenovuo J. Antibacterial activity of dental gels containing combinations of amine fluoride, stannous fluoride, and chlorhexidine against cariogenic bacteria. Scand J Dent Res 98:1–7, 1990.

Ostela I, Tenovuo J, Söderling E, Lammi E, Lammi M. Effect of chlorhexidine-sodium fluoride gel applied by tray or by toothbrush on salivary mutans streptococci. Proc Finn Dent Soc 86:9–14, 1990.

Overholser CD, Meiller TF, DePaola LG, Minah GE, Niehaus C. Comparative effects of two chemotherapeutic mouthrinses on the development of supragingival dental plaque and gingivitis. J Clin Periodontol 17:575–579, 1990.

Palcanis KG, Formica JV, Miller RA, Brooks CN, Gunsolley JC. Longitudinal evaluation of sanguinaria—Clinical and microbiological studies. Compend Contin Dent Educ (Suppl) 7:179–184, 1986.

Papapanou PN. Periodontal diseases: epidemiology. Ann Periodontol 1:1–36, 1996.

Paterson RC, Watts A, Saunders WP, Pitts NB. Modern Concepts in the Diagnosis and Treatment of Fissure Caries. London, Quintessence, 1991.

Pender N. Aspects of oral health in orthodontic patients. Br J Orthod 13:95–103, 1986.

Pendrys DG, Morse DE. Use of fluoride supplementation by children living in fluoridated communities. J Dent Child 57:343–347, 1990.

Pendrys DG, Stamm JW. Relationship of total fluoride intake to beneficial effects and enamel fluorosis. J Dent Res 69 (special issue):529–538, 1990.

Petersson LG, Maki Y, Twetman S, Edwardsson S. Mutans streptococci in saliva and interdental spaces after topical applications of an antimicrobial varnish in school-children. Oral Microbiol Immunol 6:284–287, 1991.

Persson GR, Page RC. Diagnostic characteristics of crevicular fluid aspartate aminotransferase (AST) levels associated with periodontal disease activity. J Clin Periodontol 19:43–48, 1992.

Phipps KR, Stevens VJ. Relative contribution of caries and periodontal disease in adult tooth loss for an HMO dental population. J Public Health Dent 55:250–252, 1995.

Pienihäkkinen K. Personal communication, 1990.

Pointier JP, Pine C, Jackson DL, DiDonato AK, Close J, Moore PA. Efficacy of a prebrushing rinse for orthodontic patients. Clin Prev Dent 12:12–17, 1990.

Polson AM, Reed BE. Long-term effect of orthodontic treatment on crestal alveolar bone levels. J Periodontol 55:28–34, 1984.

Poulsen S, Agerbæk N, Melsen B, Korb DC, Glavins L, Rølla G. The effect of professional toothcleaning on gingivitis and dental caries in children after 1 year. Community Dent Oral Epidemiol 4:195–199, 1976.

Poulsen S, Kirkegaard E, Bangsbo G, Bro K. Caries in clinical trial of fluoride rinses in a Danish public child dental service. Community Dent Oral Epidemiol 12:283–287, 1984.

Poulton DR. Correction of extreme deep overbite with orthodontics and orthognathic surgery. Am J Orthod Dentofac Orthop 96:275–280, 1989.

Pus MD, Way DC. Enamel loss due to orthodontic bonding with filled and unfilled resins using various clean-up techniques. Am J Orthod 77:269–283, 1980.

Quirynen M, Marechal M, Busscher HJ, Weerkamp AH, Darius PL, van Steenberghe D. The influence of surface free energy and surface roughness on early plaque formation. An in vivo study in man. J Clin Periodontol 17:138–144, 1990.

Rabe H, Miethke R-R, Magwitz A. Ergebnisse werkstoffkundlicher und mikrobiologischer Untersuchungen von sogenannten Zahnspangenreinigern. Prakt Kieferorthop 1:111–120, 1987.

Rabe H, Miethke R-R, Newesely H. Gefüge and Festigkeit von Silberloten für die Kieferorthopädie nach Behandlung mit handelsüblichen "Zahnspangenreinigern." Dtsch Zahnärztl Z 41: 714–719, 1986.

Ramfjord SP. Kieferorthopädie und parodontale Prophylaxe. In: Hösl E, Baldauf A, Diernberger R, Grosse P (eds). Kieferorthopädie und Parodontologie. Quintessenz, 723–726, 1985.

Ranney RR. Classification of periodontal diseases. Periodontol 2000 2:13–25, 1993.

Rateitschak KH. Orthodontics and periodontology. Int Dent J 18:108–120, 1968.

Reiter C, Wetzel W-E. Bearbeitung der Borstenenden bei Interdentalbürsten. Schweiz Monatsschr Zahnmed 101:431–437, 1991.

Renggli HH. Auswirkungen subgingivaler approximaler Füllungsränder auf den Entzündungsgrad der benachbarten Gingiva. Eine kleine Studie. Schweiz Monatsschr Zahnheilkd 84:1–18, 1974.

Renggli HH. Plaquehemmung durch Aminfluorid. Dtsch Zahnärztl Z 38:45–49, 1983.

Rezk-Lega F, Øgaard B, Arends J. An in vitro study on the merits of two glass ionomers for the cementation of orthodontic bands. Am J Orthod Dentofac Orthop 99:162–167, 1991.

Ripa LW. Professionally (operator) applied topical fluoride therapy: A critique. Int Dent J 31: 105–120, 1981.

Ripa LW. The roles of prophylaxes and dental prophylaxis pastes in caries prevention. In: Wei HY (ed). Clinical Use of Fluorides. Philadelphia, Lea & Febiger, 35–53, 1985.

Ripa LW. An evaluation of the use of professional (operator-applied) topical fluorides. J Dent Res 69:786–796, 1990.

Ripa LW, Leske GS, Sposato A, Varma A. Effect of prior toothcleaning on biannual professional APF topical fluoride gel-tray treatments. Results after two years. J Clin Prev Dent 5:3–7, 1983.

Rise J, Birkeland JM, Haugejorden O, Blindheim O, Furevik J. Identification of high caries risk children using prevalence of filled surfaces as a predictor variable for incidence. Community Dent Oral Epidemiol 7:340–345, 1979.

Rosenbloom RG, Tinanoff N. Salivary Stretococcus mutans levels in patients before, during and after orthodontic treatment. Am J Orthod Dentofac Orthop 100:35–37, 1991.

Roulet J-F, Roulet-Mehrens TK. The surface roughness of restorative materials and dental tissues after polishing with prophylaxis and polishing pastes. J Periodontol 53:257–266, 1982.

Rugg-Gunn AJ, MacGregor ID, Edgar WM, Ferguson MW. Toothbrushing behavior in relation to plaque and gingivitis in adolescent schoolchildren. J Periodont Res 14:231–238, 1979.

Sadowsky C, BeGole EA. Long term effects of orthodontic treatment on periodontal health. Am J Orthod 80:156–172, 1981.

Sakamaki ST, Bahn AN. Effect of orthodontic banding on localized oral lactobacilli. J Dent Res 47:275–279, 1968.

Sandham HJ, Nadeau L, Phillips HI. The effect of chlorhexidine varnish treatment on salivary mutans streptococcal levels in child orthodontic patients. J Dent Res 71:32–35, 1992.

Saxén L, Niemi M-L, Ainamo H. Intraoral spread of the antimicrobial effect of a chlorhexidine gel. Scand J Dent Res 84:304–307, 1976.

Schaeken MJ, de Haan P. Effects of sustained-release chlorhexidine acetate on the human dental plaque flora. J Dent Res 68:119–123, 1989.

Schaeken MJ, Schouten MJ, van den Kieboom CWA, van der Hoeven JS. Influence of contact time and concentration of chlorhexidine varnish on mutans streptococci in interproximal dental plaque. Caries Res 25:292–295, 1991.

Schaeken MJ, van der Hoeven JS, Hendriks JC. Effects of varnishes containing chlorhexidine on the human dental plaque flora. J Dent Res 68: 1786–1789, 1989.

Scheie AA, Arneberg P, Krogstad O. Effect of orthodontic treatment on prevalence of Streptococcus mutans in plaque and saliva. Scand J Dent Res 92:211–217, 1984.

Schiött CR, Löe H, Briner WW. Two years oral use of chlorhexidine in man. IV. Effect of various medical parameters. J Periodont Res 11: 158–164, 1976.

Schlagenhauf U, Tobien , Engelfried P. Der Einfluss kieferorthopädischer Behandlung auf Parameter des individuellen Kariesrisikos. Dtsch Zahnärztl Z 44:758–760, 1989.

Schröder F-W. Personal communication, 1992.

Schröder H. Untersuchungen zur Pathogenese der Stomatitis prothetica unter besonderer Berücksichtigung hefeähnlicher Pilze [thesis]. Free University Berlin, 1982.

Schröder U, Lindström L-G, Olsson L. Interview or questionnaire? A comparison based on the relationship between caries and dietary habits in pre-school children. Community Dent Oral Epidemiol 9:79–82, 1981.

Schulein TM, Chan DCN, Reinhardt JW. Rinsing times for a gel etchant related to enamel/composite bond strength. Gen Dent 34:296–298, 1986.

Schwartz HG. Safety profile of sanguinarine and sanguinaria extract. Compend Contin Educ Dent (Suppl) 7:212–217, 1986.

Selwitz RH, Winn DM, Kingman A, Zion GR. The prevalence of dental sealants in the US population: findings from NHANES III, 1988–1991. J Dent Res 75:652–660, 1996.

Seppä L, Hausen H. Die Identifizierung von Kariesrisikopatienten. Eine Übersicht. Oralprophylaxe 10:96–107, 1988a.

Seppä L, Hausen H. Frequency of initial caries lesions as predictor of future caries increment in children. Scand J Dent Res 96:9–13, 1988b.

Seppä L, Hausen H, Luoma H. Relationship between caries and fluoride uptake by enamel from two fluoride varnishes in a community with fluoridated water. Caries Res 16:404–412, 1982.

Seppä L, Hausen H, Pöllänen L, Helasharju K, Kärkkäinen S. Past caries recordings made in public dental clinics as predictors of caries prevalence in early adolescence. Community Dent Oral Epidemiol 17:277–281, 1989.

Seppä L, Pöllänen L. Caries preventive effect of two fluoride varnishes and a fluoride mouthrinse. Caries Res 21:375–379, 1987.

Seppä L, Tolonen T. Caries preventive effect of fluoride varnish applications performed two or four times a year. Scand J Dent Res 98:102–105, 1990.

Seymour RA, Heasman PA. Tetracyclines in the management of periodontal diseases. A review. J Clin Periodontol 22:22–35, 1995.

Shannon IL. Prevention of decalcification in orthodontic patients. J Clin Orthod 15:694–705, 1981.

Shaw WC, Addy M, Ray C. Dental and social effects of malocclusion and effectiveness of orthodontic treatment—A review. Community Dent Oral Epidemiol 8:36–45, 1980.

Shaw WC, Gabe MJ, Jones BM. The expectations of orthodontic patients in South Wales and St. Louis, Missouri. Br J Orthod 6:203–205, 1979.

Shaw WC, Humphreys S. Influence of children's dentofacial appearance on teacher expectations. Community Dent Oral Epidemiol 10:313–319, 1982.

Sheiham A. Prevention and control of periodontal disease. International Conference on Research in the Biology of Periodontal Disease. Chicago, University of Illinois, 309–368, 1977.

Silness J, Roynstrand T. Relationship between alignment conditions of teeth in anterior segments and dental health. J Clin Periodontol 12:312–320, 1985.

Silverstein S, Gold S, Heilbron D, Nehus D, Wycoff S. Effect of supervised deplaquing on dental caries, gingivitis and plaque. J Dent Res 56:abstract 85, 1977.

Silverstone LM. State of the art on sealant research and priorities for further research. J Dent Educ 48:107–118, 1984.

Silverstone LM, Wefel JS, Zimmerman BF, Clarkson BH, Featherstone MJ. Remineralization of natural and artificial lesions in human dental enamel. Caries Res 15:138–157, 1981.

Simonsen RJ. Retention and effectiveness of dental sealant after 15 years. J Am Dent Assoc 122:34–42, 1991.

Simonsen RJ. Glass ionomer as fissure sealant—a critical review. J Public Health Dent 56:146–149; discussion 161–163, 1996.

Singh SM. Efficacy of a prebrushing rinse in reducing dental plaque. Am J Dent 3:15–16, 1990.

Skjörland KK. Plaque accumulation on different dental filling materials. Scand J Dent Res 81:538–542, 1973.

Slavkin HC. First encounters: transmission of infectious oral diseases from mother to child. J Am Dent Assoc 128:773–778, 1997.

Slots J, Rams TE: Antibiotics in periodontal therapy: Advantages and disadvantages. J Clin Periodontol 17:479–493, 1990.

Sluiter JB, Purdell-Lewis DJ. Lower fluoride concentrations for topical application. Caries Res 18:56–62, 1984.

Smith BA, Shanbour GS, Caffesse RG, Morrison EC, Dennison JD. In vitro polishing effectiveness of interdental aids on root surfaces. J Clin Periodontol 13:597–603, 1986.

Snyder JA, McVay JT, Brown FH, Stoffers KW, Harvey RC, Houston GD, Patrissi GA. The effect of air abrasive polishing on blood pH and electrolyte concentrations in healthy mongrel dogs. J Periodontol 61:81–86, 1990.

Socransky SS. Caries-susceptibility tests. Ann NY Acad Sci 153:137–146, 1968.

Söder PÖ, Frithiof L, Söder B. Spirochaetes and granulocytes at sites involved in periodontal disease. Arch Oral Biol 35:197S–200S, 1990.

Sonis AL, Snell W. An evaluation of a fluoride-releasing, visible light-activated bonding system for orthodontic bracket placement. Am J Orthod Dentofac Orthop 95:306–311, 1989.

Southard GL, Boulware RT, Walborn DR, Groznik WJ, Thorne EE, Yankell SL. Sanguinarine, a new antiplaque agent. Retention and plaque specificity. J Am Dent Assoc 108: 338–341, 1984.

Southard MS, Cohen ME, Ralls SA, Rouse LA. Effects of fixed-appliance orthodontic treatment on caries indices. Am J Orthod Dentofac Orthop 90:122–126, 1986.

Spurrier SW, Hall SH, Joondeph DR, Shapiro PS, Riedel RA. A comparison of apical tooth resorption during orthodontic treatment in endodontically treated and vital teeth. Am J Orthod Dentofacial Orthop 97:130–134, 1990.

Stecksén-Blicks C. Salivary counts of lactobacilli and Streptococcus mutans in caries prediction. Scand J Dent Res 93:204–212, 1985.

Stephan RM. Intra-oral hydrogen-ion concentrations associated with dental caries activity. J Dent Res 23:257–266, 1944.

Stephen KW, Russell JI, Creanor SL, Burchell CH. Comparison of fibre optic transillumination and radiographic caries diagnosis. Community Dent Oral Epidemiol 12:90–94, 1987.

Stookey GK. Critical evaluation of the composition and use of topical fluorides. J Dent Res 69:805–812, 1990.

Stookey GK, Schemehorn BR. A method for assessing the relative abrasion of prophylaxis materials. J Dent Res 58:588–592, 1978.

Sturzenberger OP, Leonard GJ. The effect of a mouthwash as an adjunct in tooth cleaning. J Periodontol 40:299–301, 1969.

Suhonen J, Tenovuo J. Neue Wege in der Kariesprävention. Phillip J 5:279–286, 1989.

Svanberg ML, Loesche WJ. Implantation of Streptococcus mutans on tooth surfaces in man. Arch Oral Biol 23:551–556, 1978.

Svanbom DD, Davison CO. Crevicular delivery of sanguinaria to control gingivitis. J Am Dent Assoc 114:591–594, 1987.

Svatun B, Saxton CA, Huntington E, Cummins D. The effects of three silica dentifrices containing triclosan on supragingival plaque and calculus formation and on gingivitis. Int Dent J 43: 441–452, 1993.

Taylor GW, Burt BA, Becker MP, Genco RJ, Shlossman M, Knowler WC, Pettitt DJ. Severe periodontitis and risk for poor glycemic control in patients with non-insulin-dependent diabetes mellitus. J Periodontol 67:1085–1093, 1996.

Tell RT, Sydiskis RJ, Isaacs RD, Davidson WM. Long-term cytotoxicity of orthodontic direct-bonding adhesives. Am J Orthod Dentofac Orthop 93:419–422, 1988.

ten Cate JM, Jongbloed WL, Arends J. Remineralization of artificial enamel lesions in vitro. Caries Res 15:60–69, 1981.

Tenovuo J, Häkkinen P, Paunio P, Emilson CG. Effects of chlorhexidine-fluoride gel treatments in mothers on the establishment of mutans streptococci in primary teeth and the development of dental caries in children. Caries Res 26: 275–280, 1992.

Thilander B, Nyman S, Karring T, Magnusson I. Bone regeneration in alveolar bone dehiscences related to orthodontic tooth movements. Eur J Orthod 5:105–114, 1983.

Thompson RE, Way DC. Enamel loss due to prophylaxis and multiple bonding/debonding of orthodontic attachments. Am J Orthod 79: 282–295, 1981.

Twetman S, Petersson LG. Effect of different chlorhexidine varnish regimens on mutans streptococci levels in interdental plaque and saliva. Caries Res 31:189–193, 1997.

Thorstensson H, Kuylenstierna J, Hugoson A. Medical status and complications in relation to periodontal disease experience in insulin-dependent diabetics. J Clin Periodontol 23:194–202, 1996.

Underwood ML, Rawls HR, Zimmerman BF. Clinical evaluation of a fluoride-exchanging resin as an orthodontic adhesive. Am J Orthod Dentofacial Orthop 96:93–99, 1989.

Valk JWP, Duijsters PPE, ten Cate JM, Davidson CL. The long-term retention and effectiveness of APF and neutral KF fluoridation agents on sound and etched bovine enamel. Caries Res 19:46–52, 1985.

Vanarsdall RL. Complications of orthodontic treatment. Curr Opin Dent 1:622–633, 1991.

van de Rijke JW. Use of dyes in cariology. Int Dent J 41:111–116, 1991.

van der Velden U, van der Weijden GA, Jansen-Danser M, Nijboer A, Timmermann M. Klinische Studie zur Wirksamkeit des Plaque-Entferners Braun Plak Control (D 5) im Vergleich zu einer herkömmlichen elektrischen Zahnbürste (Braun D 3) und einer manuellen Zahnbürste. Manufacturer's information, Braun 1991.

van der Weijden GA, Danser MM, Nijboer A, Timmermann MF, van der Velden U. The plaque-removing efficacy of an oscillating/rotating toothbrush. A short-term study. J Clin Periodontol 20:273–278, 1993a.

van der Weijden GA, Timmerman MF, Nijboer A, Lie MA, van der Velden U. A comparative study of electric toothbrushes for the effectiveness of plaque removal in relation to toothbrushing duration. J Clin Periodontol 20:476–481, 1993b.

van der Weijden GA, Timmermann MF, Rejerse E, Danser MM, Mantel MS, Nijboer A, van der Velden U. The long-term effect of an oscillating/rotating electric toothbrush on gingivitis. An 8-month clinical study. J Clin Periodontol 21:139–145, 1994.

van Dijken JW, Sjöström S, Wing K. The effect of different types of composite resin filling materials on marginal gingiva. J Clin Periodontol 14:185–189, 1987.

van Rijkom HM, Truin GJ, van't Hof MA. A meta-analysis of clinical studies on the caries-inhibiting effect of chlorhexidine treatment. J Dent Res 75:790–795, 1996.

Varrela J. Occurrence of malocclusion in attritive environment—a study of a skull sample from southwest Finland. Scand J Dent Res 98:242–247, 1990.

Verdonschot EH, Bronkhorst EM, Burgersdijk RCW, König KG, Schaeken MJM, Truin GJ. Performance of some diagnostic systems in examinations for small occlusal carious lesions. Caries Res 26:59–64, 1992.

Vestergaard V, Moss A, Pedersen HO, Poulsen S. The effect of supervised tooth cleansing every second week on dental caries in Danish school children. Acta Odontol Scand 36:249–252, 1978.

Viazis AD, DeLong R, Bevis RR, Douglas WH, Speidel TM. Enamel surface abrasion from ceramic orthodontic brackets: A special case report. Am J Orthod Dentofac Orthop 96:514–518, 1989.

Waerhaug J. The interdental brush and its place in operative and crown and bridge dentistry. J Oral Rehabil 3:107–113, 1976.

Wagner MJ, Tvrdy JL, Barnes GP, Lyon TC, Parker WA. Sodium retention from mouthwashes. Clin Prev Dent 11:3–6, 1989.

Walker JD, Jensen ME, Pinkham JR. A clinical review of preventive resin restorations. J Dent Child 57:257–259, 1990.

Wallmann C, Krasse B. A simple method for monitoring mutans streptococci in margins of restorations. J Dent 21:216–219, 1993.

Wang WN, Sheen DH. The effect of pretreatment with fluoride on the tensile strength of orthodontic bonding. Angle Orthod 61:31–34, 1991.

Weaks LM, Lescher NB, Barnes CM, Holroyd SV. Clinical evaluation of the Prophy-Jet as an instrument for routine removal of tooth stain and plaque. J Periodontol 55:486–488, 1984.

Weerheijm KL, de Soet JJ, van Amerongen WE, de Graaff J. Sealing of occlusal hidden caries lesions: an alternative for curative treatment? ASDC J Dent Child 59:263–268, 1992

Wennström JL, Heijl L, Dahlen G, Gröndahl K. Periodic subgingival antimicrobial irrigation of periodontal pockets. I. Clinical observations. J Clin Periodontol 14:541–550, 1987.

White BA, Antczak BA, Weinstein MC. Issues in the economic evaluation of community water fluoridation. J Dent Educ 53:646–657, 1989.

Widenheim J. A time-related study of intake patterns of fluoride tablets among Swedish preschool children and parental attitudes. Community Dent Oral Epidemiol 10:196–300, 1982.

Wikner S. An attempt to motivate improved sugar discipline in a 12-year-old high caries-risk group. Community Dent Oral Epidemiol 14:5–7, 1986.

Wilcoxon DB, Ackerman RJ, Killoy WJ, Love JW, Sakumura JS, Tira DE: The effectiveness of a counterrotational-action power toothbrush on plaque control and gingival health in orthodontic patients. Am J Orthod Dentofac Orthop 99: 7–14, 1991.

Williams P, Fenwick A, Schou L, Adams W. A clinical trial of an orthodontic toothbrush. Eur J Orthod 9:295–304, 1987.

Wilson RF, Ashley FP. Identification of caries risk in schoolchildren: Salivary buffering capacity and bacterial counts, sugar intake and caries experience as predictors of 2-year and 3-year caries increment. Br Dent J 166:99–102, 1989.

World Health Organization (WHO). Appropriate Use of Fluorides for Human Health. Geneva, WHO, 1986.

World Health Organization. Fluorides and oral health. Technical Report Series, no. 846, 1994.

World Health Organization/Borrow Dental Milk Foundation. Symposium I: International milk fluoridation projects. Presented at The 4th World Congress on Preventive Dentistry, Umeå, Sweden, 1993.

Yankell SL, Emling RC, Cohen DW, Vanarsdall RJ. A four-week evaluation of oral health in orthodontic patients using a new plaque-removal device. Compend Contin Educ Dent (Suppl) 6: 123–127, 1985.

Yeung SD, Howell S, Fahey P. Oral hygiene program for orthodontic patients. Am J Orthod Dentofacial Orthop 96:208–213, 1989.

Youngblood JJ, Killoy WJ, Love JW, Drisko C. Effectiveness of a new home-plaque removal instrument in removing subgingival and interproximal plaque—A preliminary in vivo report. Compend Contin Educ Dent (Suppl) 6:128–132, 1985.

Zachrisson BU. Oral hygiene for orthodontic patients. Current concepts and practical advice. Am J Orthod 66:487–497, 1974.

Zachrisson BU. Fluoride application procedures in orthodontic practice—Current concepts. Angle Orthod 45:72–81, 1975.

Zachrisson BU. Cause and prevention of injuries to teeth and supporting structures during orthodontic treatment. Am J Orthod 69:285–300, 1976.

Zachrisson BU. Clinical experience with direct bonded orthodontic retainers. Am J Orthod 71: 440–448, 1977.

Zachrisson BU, Alnæs L. Periodontal condition in orthodontically treated and untreated individuals. I. Loss of attachment, gingival pocket depth and clinical crown height. Angle Orthod 43:402–412, 1973.

Zachrisson BU, Brobakken BO. Clinical comparison of direct versus indirect bonding with different bracket types and adhesives. Am J Orthod 74:66–78, 1978.

Zachrisson BU, Skogan Ö, Höymyhr S. Enamel cracks in debonded, debanded, and orthodontically untreated teeth. Am J Orthod 77:307–319, 1980.

Zachrisson S, Zachrisson BU. Caries incidence and orthodontic treatment with fixed appliances. Scand J Dent Res 79:183–192, 1971.

Zachrisson S, Zachrisson BU. Gingival condition associated with orthodontic treatment. Angle Orthod 41:26–34, 1972.

Zickert I, Emilson CG, Krasse B. Effect of caries preventive measures in children highly infected with bacterium Streptococcus mutans. Arch Oral Biol 27:861–868, 1982.

Zyskind K, Zyskind D, Duncker M, Miethke R-R, Steinberg D, Friedman M. Eine Neue Methode zur Inhibition von Plaque-Akkumulation bei Kindern mit herausnehmbaren kieferorthopädischen Geräten. Prakt Kieferorthop 4:53–58, 1990.

Index